by Marshall de Graffenried Ruffin, MD, MPH, MBA, CPE, FACPE

# Digital Doctors

**American College of Physician Executives**
4890 West Kennedy Boulevard, Suite 200
Tampa, Florida 33609
813/287-2000

Copyright 1999 by Marshall Ruffin Jr., MD, MPH, MBA, CPE, FACPE.
All rights reserved. Reproduction or translation of this work beyond that permitted by applicable copyright law without the permission of the author is prohibited. Requests for permission to reprint or for further information should be directed to the Permissions Editor, ACPE, Two Urban Centre, Suite 200, 4890 West Kennedy Boulevard, Tampa, Florida 33609.

ISBN: 0-924674-63-6
Library of Congress Card Number: 98-89673

Printed in the United States of America by Hillsboro Printing Company, Tampa, Florida

# Foreword

Marshall Ruffin has been "spreading the digital gospel" to physicians who wish to lead for about a decade now. While the details of the message are in constant flux, given the rapidity of change in the high-world of computers and informatics, the overarching rationale has remained firm. We live in digital times, and our lives are apt to become more and more dominated by the digital revolution. Nothing, I think, speaks more eloquently of this historical force than a new publication entitled *Time Digital*. The venerable *Time* magazine has spun its news coverage of matters digital into a freestanding monthly.

In this collection of essays based on a series that has been running in *Physician Executive* for the past 6-7 years, Dr. Ruffin updates and expands on his contention that, to lead the health care delivery system, physicians will have to acknowledge and understand the power and scope of digital information. They will have to become conversant with both the concepts of informatics and their application in the work-a-day health care world.

And that is what this book is most wonderfully about—the vastness of informatics' contributions to improvements in the ways in which health care services are delivered. This is no ivory tower treatise. But it may qualify as a paean. Dr. Ruffin believes in the power of informatics to transform health care delivery, bringing it back, as he states it, to "managing care." Even if you do not totally agree with all the positions Dr. Ruffin takes, you must admire the enthusiasm and drive that he brings to this subject. And you will walk away from this book a little more convinced that your future is digital and a lot better armed to deal with it.

**Wesley Curry**
*Managing Editor, Book Publishing*
American College of Physician Executives
November 1998

# Preface

After I read the book *Being Digital,* by Nicholas Negroponte, I began writing the chapters of this book, musing on the implications of being digital for health care in general and for the work of physicians in particular. You owe yourself the experience of reading *Being Digital* (see chapter 2). Unlike most in academe, Dr. Negroponte writes with humor and enthusiasm about the implications of the digital revolution happening all around us. He explains well the meaning of being digital and managing information in digital form. His optimism is infectious.

I hope this book helps you to consider the myriad ways in which digital computers and communication technology can help you do your job better. You may be a physician or a nurse. You may be an administrator of a hospital or a group practice. You may be a manager of a health plan; a physician hospital organization (PHO); a medical service organization (MSO); a preferred provider organization (PPO); or an other weird arrangement (OWA) of physicians, hospitals, and insurers. Whatever your role, the ineluctable progress of technological improvement, with simultaneously declining prices and improving productivity, will lead you frequently to look for ways of deploying these technologies to offset payroll costs and to improve the operations of your organization.

Functions of digital information systems that were not thinkable five years ago are thinkable today, affordable tomorrow, and commonplace the day after tomorrow. We may overestimate the short-term implications of new technologies, but we tend to underestimate the long-term implications of those same technologies. The automobile did not replace horses as quickly as early enthusiasts predicted, but it brought with it highways, interstate travel, suburbs, and fast food that no one predicted when the automobile first became available. Did you think that you would have accurate voice recognition on your PC when you bought your first PC in the mid-1980s? When you bought your first 1200-baud modem not so long ago, did you think that your telephone line would one day carry a digital stream of data at five megabits per second? Did you ever think you'd be considering a computer-based patient record for your office practice when you installed your first practice management system? Did you think when you made your first house call that your patients in the late 1990s would discuss their symptoms and allow you to examine them by video teleconference from their homes to your office? Did you think when you finished medical school that, one day in the late 1990s, insurers, employers, and government agencies would collect data from your patients and develop a report card on your practice habits?

In this book we will discuss these improbable eventualities that have become reality. We tend to overestimate the immediate consequences of new technologies and underestimate their long-term effects. Some pundits proclaim the imminent arrival of hospitals on wristwatches. Less inclined to vague futurism, I have limited my predictions to applications of digital information management technology that I think will be available to you in less than five years. Most of the technologies to which I refer are available today. Your job is to consider them in light of your plans for your practice, hospital, health plan, or delivery system and to decide which you should consider adding to the processes of information management your organization uses now.

I want to thank Wes Curry and Susan Sasenick, my able editors at the American College of Physician Executives, who edited most of the chapters in this book when they were articles in *Physician Executive* magazine.

My wife, Paula Thomas Ruffin, deserves special thanks for giving me the inspiration to publish my thoughts and having the patience to wait for me to finish.

**Marshall Ruffin Jr., MD, MPH, MBA, CPE, FACPE**
Charlottesville, Virginia
November 1998

# Introduction

Advances in information technology are helping clinicians to realize the promise of "scientific medicine," which includes systematic study of available medical research on specific clinical situations, benchmarking, outcomes monitoring, predictive modeling, and clinical pathways. The practice of scientific medicine requires integration of individual clinical expertise and the best available clinical research. Using scientific medicine, clinicians can apply the disciplines and techniques of clinical research to their practice of medicine, one patient at a time.

Scientific medicine, practiced by individual clinicians, enables organizations to implement continuous clinical quality improvement programs. Previously, such programs have struggled when there has been a lack of clinically meaningful data needed to establish benchmarks, measure variation in clinical practices, and monitor compliance with generally accepted clinical processes and clinical results.

Standards, open information systems, data warehouses, and medical knowledge bases, including electronic access to the National Library of Medicine, help clinicians in a health care delivery system practice scientific medicine. They need technical infrastructure, decision-making processes, analytical skills, clinical databases, and predictive models and clinical pathways to standardize and rationalize clinical care among physicians. The health care system will profile the practice habits of physicians for managed care contracting and for continuous clinical quality improvement.

Progress in medical care begins with a hypothesis posed by a clinician, manager, or research scientist that is followed by one or more clinical research trials to test the validity of the hypothesis:

- "I wonder if this medication will improve survival of patients with these characteristics?" or
- "I wonder if this surgical procedure will improve function in these patients?"

To answer those questions, detailed information about patients is recorded, stored in computers, and analyzed with appropriate statistical techniques to identify variation in the outcomes of patients that can be attributed to variation in treatment, and not to random variation alone.

The treatment choices of individual physicians, human nature being what it is, are more influenced by the recent experience of the physician with individual patients than by clinical research results. For most physicians in practice, medicine has a human face; it is not about populations and statistics. There are no clinical trials to tell a physician how to treat his own patients, because the clinical trials are based on patients other than his. But you cannot determine if one treatment is better than another from individual cases. Using scientific medicine, however, individual physicians can apply the disciplines and results of clinical research to their practice of medicine, one patient at a time.

Duke University Medical Center leads the nation in scientific medical care for heart disease. Eugene Stead, MD, then the Chairman of Medicine at Duke, determined in the 1970s that Duke should build an electronic medical record and data warehouse for the systematic study of the treatments and outcomes of all patients with heart disease. Duke created the Cardiovascular Databank,[1] which has evolved into a massive information system. Yearly, Duke collects more than 70,000 detailed, structured forms on the history, physical examinations, and laboratory studies of patients with heart disease, as well as forms defining the results of surgical procedures, medical treatments, and the outcomes of patients.

Dr. Robert M. Califf, a cardiologist on the faculty of Duke University Medical Center who directs the Duke Cardiovascular Databank, said of medical diagnosis and treatment of patients with heart disease before the Databank was available: "The old system was one in which physicians studied the chemistry and physiology of how a disease worked and implemented theories based on this. Care was based on the physician's own observations, and training was essentially an apprenticeship. But you can't decide if a therapy is working or not based on each individual case. Now we have the computer to remember and aggregate numbers. We can measure what happened to patients, and if it wasn't successful, we can change our approach. We can give multiple examples of where what we thought was right was in fact dead wrong."[2]

In the future, with the advent of managed care competition and the growing importance of standardized, efficient, and effective care, private health care organizations will invest in standardized data collection in electronic form and sophisticated predictive modeling of patients' characteristics to predict their outcomes.

Professionals predict the future for a living. Every physician is paid to predict the future. A physician determines a diagnosis, a prognosis and a course of treatment for a patient based on the best information he can collect on his patient, his understanding of the specific condition, and his training and experience. Predictive modeling is a new tool that a physician can use to determine the likely outcomes of different treatments for a patient, based on the patient's own condition. Using this tool, the physician and his patient can select a treatment based on the highest likelihood of the desired outcome.[3-6]

The technology for predictive modeling is maturing at a rapid rate with the advent of sophisticated mathematical techniques for pattern recognition (the new "intermaths"—regression analysis, Monte Carlo simulations, neural networks, and genetic algorithms) and parallel processing computers. A recently published book, *After Thought* by James Bailey, speaks elegantly to these trends.[7] Bailey argues that mathematics has matured from the study of place (geometry and navigation), through the study of pace (algebra and calculus), to the current study of complex *patterns* in large data sets using computers (predictive modeling).

# Introduction vii

Bailey and other proponents of the new intermaths believe that static equations do not have the subtlety and accuracy to model complex biological processes well and accurately predict the outcomes of medical treatment. A neural network recently proved best in predicting one-year mortality rates for patients with heart failure, using data from echocardiograms to make its predictions, compared to clinical judgment of cardiologists, linear discriminant analysis, and automatic heuristic methods.[8] Neural networks can accurately diagnosis patients with glaucoma using data from automated visual field studies and structural data from computerized image analysis.[9] Neural networks perform well in predicting patients with acute appendicitis.[10]

Predictive modeling provides powerful tools to help clinicians evaluate patients and select treatment protocols. For example, Dr. Eric Peterson at the Duke Clinical Research Institute, which maintains the Duke Cardiovascular Databank, has developed models for physicians to use in their practices. "After initial consultation with a patient complaining of chest pain, the physician can look at a model which incorporates this information and his patient's vital statistics-such as age, weight and other health factors-to help him determine the next course of action. If the model shows that the patient might have a high likelihood of having a serious problem, the physician may then decide to skip what is typically the next step, a treadmill test, and move on to a higher level," Peterson said. At each successive stage, the physician can consult a new model to help direct his decision-making. Peterson said he uses the models a great deal in his work. "Most patients in the 1990s are very involved with their care and want to participate in the decisions," he said. "They appreciate knowing the relative successes of different treatments. Knowing the specific benefits and risks of a treatment, we can make a plan that we both become very comfortable with."[1]

Scientific medicine and continuous clinical quality improvement have been given a big boost recently by the Joint Commission on Accreditation of Healthcare Organizations (JCAHO). Under JCAHO's ORYX Initiative, health care providers are now required to implement effective outcomes measurement processes. JCAHO has established a central role for itself in building a "national quality oversight system" built on four pillars: "The *first pillar* will be an adaptable standards-based evaluation framework that credibly relates sound processes to good patient outcomes and effectively reduces risk in the delivery of care. The *second pillar* will be a group of mature, user-friendly, cost-effective, useful measurement systems.

"The *third pillar* will be the capability to evaluate, in a substantive fashion, all levels of the delivery system, from the individual practitioner's office to the complex integrated delivery system, and thereby be able to provide reassurances to the public about the quality of care being provided across the country. The *fourth pillar* will be achievement of consensus on the best evaluation tools and effective coordination of evaluation activities among all major evaluators in the private and public sectors."[11]

At its January 1997 board meeting, JCAHO approved the plan and timetable for integrating the use of outcomes and other performance measures into the accreditation process. "By December 31, 1997, each accredited hospital and long-term care organization must select (or already be participating in) one or more performance measurement systems that have been accepted by the Joint Commission. Also by December 31, 1997, each accredited hospital and long-term care organization must select from its performance measurement system(s)—for future reporting purposes—at least two clinical measures that relate to at least 20 percent of its patient or resident population. Each accredited organization will be asked to provide to the Joint Commission the identity of its performance measurement system(s) and the clinical measures it has selected by December 31, 1997.

"Finally, each accredited hospital and long term-care organization will be required to begin submitting data to the Joint Commission relative to its selected measures no later than the first quarter of 1999. Because the Joint Commission will need comparative data for monitoring purposes, it is expected that actual data submissions will be performed by the participating performance measurement systems."[11]

Clinicians and administrators need to learn the effects of clinical decisions, based on systematic retrospective analysis of clinical and administrative data. Clinical data warehouses represent valuable resources for retrospective analysis for education, predictive modeling, benchmarks, outcomes improvement, marketing, and administration.[12,13]

Standards for data collected across encounters and over time are critical for health care organizations if they are to pool data, establish benchmarks and norms, and share clinical data with collaborating organizations.[14] These processes, enabled by data standards, are essential for:

- Practicing scientific medicine.

- Implementing an effective outcome measurement process, as required by the ORYX Initiative.

The speed and skill with which an organization adjusts to changes in its business environment determine its success in the marketplace. As with organisms, the ability to learn quickly and incisively marks organizations that grow and prosper in rapidly changing times. Most health care delivery systems are natural laboratories for study and improvement in the health care of people and the medical care of patients. Health care systems need to invest in continuing education of their clinicians, using data and information they glean from the care of their own patients and health plan members. No academic research trials can come close in number of subjects under study to the numbers of health plan members and patients whose health care is influenced directly by health care delivery systems. Health care systems have an opportunity, some would say an obligation, to invest resources in standardized data collection and training of their clinical and managerial leaders to analyze those data to find opportunities for clinical quality improvement. We can only hope they will see the opportunity they have to systematically study and improve care and, in the process, develop considerable competitive advantage in the marketplace for their services.

In 1990, Peter Senge published his extraordinarily successful book entitled *The Fifth Discipline, The Art & Practice of the Learning Organization.*[15] Learning organizations build intellectual capital. Since 1996, a number of influential books have appeared on the subject of intellectual capital.[16-18] Some corporations have begun to calculate and report to investors their investment in intellectual capital.[19] Intellectual capital represents the knowledge of an organization that helps it compete for business and grow profitably. When the common stocks of companies trade at substantial premiums to their book values, the market is valuing the likely stream of future earnings that are due to assets that are not reflected on the balance sheets of those companies. In the information age, companies are valued on the basis

# Introduction

of the talent they employ, their effectiveness in using that talent, their ability to learn from and satisfy their customers, and their ability to innovate and change.

Steward has a good definition of intellectual capital: "By 'intellectual capital' I don't mean intellectual property (such as patients and copyrights), though that is one part of intellectual capital. Intellectual capital is the sum of everything everybody in a company knows that gives it a competitive edge. Unlike the assets with which business people and accountants are familiar—land, factories, equipment, cash—intellectual capital is intangible. It is the knowledge of a workforce: the training and intuition of a team of chemists who discover a billion-dollar new drug or the know-how of workmen who come up with a thousand different ways to improve the efficiency of a factory. It is the electronic network that transports information at light speed through a company, so that it can react to the market faster than its rivals. It is the collaboration—the shared learning—between a company and its customers, which forges a bond between them that brings the customer back again and again.

"In a sentence: Intellectual capital is intellectual material—knowledge, information, intellectual property, experience—that can be put to use to create wealth. It is collective brainpower. It's hard to identify and harder still to deploy effectively. But once you find it and exploit it, you win."[16]

Most health care systems represent a learning laboratory of hundreds of medical organizations, including thousands of clinicians caring for hundreds of thousands of health plan members and patients. Some, such as Kaiser Permanente and the military health care systems, treat millions of people. Most health care systems need to establish a culture of one health care system with shared data standards, but most act like collections of disparate facilities with few, if any, common information systems. As such, most health care systems need standardized digital databases and networks (what Stewart calls the structural capital component of intellectual capital) to collect, store, and analyze data about the processes and outcomes of care of its member facilities and medical groups. They need standardized and shared clinical and administrative data dictionaries, medical record numbering schemes, charge masters, and cost accounting methods.

Most health care systems need a model for sharing knowledge across the enterprise and with the outside world, fostering learning by health care system clinicians and enhancing the value of the health care system for them. Most health care systems need to establish the means and incentives for clinicians to communicate among themselves clinical insights for producing better financial and clinical outcomes for their patients. A clinical guideline developed in a health care system hospital in Arizona that reduces the complications of patients with diabetes should be shared throughout the health care system. A disease management program employed in southern California that saves lives should be shared within all of the health care systems and published for the world.

There exists a rich literature now of journal articles and books on the measurable cost-effectiveness of scientific medicine and continuing education. For instance:

- Automated pharmaceutical inventory systems for hospitals help hospital formulary committees use cost-effectiveness analysis, peer review, and continuing medical education to influence the purchase of drugs by hospitals and physicians' prescribing habits in ways beneficial to patients and the financial condition of the hospital.[20]

- Nurses offered continuing professional education relevant to their work have higher morale and work more efficiently that those deprived of such applicable instruction.[21]

- Hospital administrators, with the leadership of physician executives, can and have developed successful continuing education programs to promote cost-effective physician behavior that benefits their hospitals financially—based on educational display of the variation in their practice habits and emphasis on scientific medicine.[22]

- Quality improvement programs in hospitals can reduce hospital charges and, in the era of capitation, lead to long-term financial stability for hospitals and health care systems.[23]

- Cost-benefit analysis of educational programs for general practitioners in Sweden on prevention and treatment of depression led to measurable net savings (after expenses) to Swedish society of $26 million.[24]

- Inexpensive and readily available quantitative methods can give impressive information to physicians that leads to substantial changes in their drug prescription patterns and saves resources without injuring patients in any way.[25]

- Scientific medicine offers strategies and techniques of observational data analysis that support medical progress without requiring randomized clinical trials.[26] There are identifiable costs and benefits of relying on observational data analysis in large clinical databases to determine clinical policies instead of relying solely on the results of randomized clinical trials.

- Many circumstances now justify developing clinical policies from analysis of observational data—scientific medicine—in carefully developed and validated clinical data warehouses.[27] Scientific medicine can be seen as an acceptable, even necessary, limitation of clinical freedom, because it leads to practice guidelines meant to standardize and reduce variation in clinical care.

- It is clear that costs of care must be considered in evaluation of clinical policies because there are known situations in which marginally beneficial services to patients clearly are not affordable if made available to all patients who might benefit from them. As health care systems move from fee-for-service medicine to capitation, these analyses will become more common and acceptable to clinicians.[28]

- Health authorities successfully are using some of the techniques of scientific medicine, clinical audits, and clinical guidelines to promote clinical cost-effectiveness in the context of contracts that place health authorities at financial risk for the care of populations of patients over time.[29] Audits of the practice habits of busy community physicians can compare the effectiveness and the efficiency of those physicians to standards established by "scientific medicine."

- Quantitative methods can calculate the benefits to patients of changes in idiosyncratic practice habits to those supported by generally accepted clinical guidelines. Efficiency and appropriateness of clinical practice can be measured with observational data analysis.[30]

- Clinicians trained in clinical care and health services research (biostatistics and epidemiology) need to lead implementation of clinical practice audits and scientific medicine programs and to mediate between clinicians and managers to achieve optimal cost-effective care. Otherwise, the beneficial and cost-effective role of practice guidelines may be subverted by administrative fiat of health care commissioners whose purpose is first to reduce costs and second to improve care.[31]

# Introduction

Most health care systems need to focus on improving the operations of health care system facilities and affiliated medical groups through continuing education. With a focus on clinical operations, a health care system can make continuing education more immediately relevant to physicians and beneficial to the organization; and it will be more immediately valuable to the health care system. What do we mean by focusing continuing education on the operations of the health care system? We mean teaching physicians about variation in care that exists among the health care system clinicians, based on real, observational data sets (claims, laboratory results, and pharmaceutical orders).

Various committees of clinicians within the health care system are promulgating clinical guidelines. To expedite and enhance their work, the health care system can:

- Develop research that shows the need for and value of those guidelines.
- Calculate predicted outcomes from implementing those guidelines.
- Measure the effects of those guidelines over time.
- Teach physicians to understand the data, the analyses, and the guidelines and how to implement them.

A web site is an excellent vehicle to disseminate the work and insights gleaned from analysis of data for continuing education. Most health care systems would do themselves and their customers a favor by:

- Creating a catapult web site to useful educational content for continuing medical education of health care system physicians. This minimizes the amount health care systems must invest in educational content, but gives health care system physicians a simple and efficient way to find educational content on the Web. The catapult site should be organized by medical specialty.

- Identifying experts within the health care system in various specialties and have them moderate discussion of clinical cases posted by health care system physicians. This will establish the culture of the health care system as one organization without walls rather than a collection of disparate facilities and will promote the value of the health care system as a source of knowledge for its regions and constituent facilities.

- Beginning analysis of observational data from the health care system, developing tutorials designed to teach physicians about the findings, and posting the tutorials and findings on the web site. From the tutorials and findings will flow interest in clinical guidelines. The analyses can be used to justify pilot studies of guidelines. The results of pilot studies of guidelines can be posted on the web site and can help promote the adoption of successful guidelines that lead to improvement in clinical and financial outcomes of care.

Technologies for analysis of data and dissemination of the contents of continuing education are readily available. Administrative and clinical data about the care of patients within the health care system can be made anonymous to protect individuals' privacy and then pooled into large comparative databases so epidemiologists and health data analysts can search for measurable variation in the care of similar patients within the organization. Significant variation—once found, publicized, and addressed—is an opportunity for quality improvement. Distance learning technologies—CD-ROM, video conferencing, the World Wide Web—are readily available, are inexpensive to deploy, and reduce the cost of disseminating insights into ways to improve clinical processes of care throughout the health care system.

Care management programs, developing now in many health care organizations, introduce to managers and clinicians methods and technologies to standardize care processes and improve outcomes for patients and health plan members. Managed care should mean managing care, which is more than negotiating discounts from providers and forcing them to obtain prior approval for referrals. Managing care means measuring care and responding to the measurement with process changes to improve care.

Most care management programs include substantial investment in information technologies. They collect data about the care rendered to patients, inform clinicians at the point of care about a patient's medical record and about practice guidelines that might apply to that patient, and store data in data warehouses for retrospective observational data analysis.

The technologies for relational database management and online analytical processing continue to improve, and the costs of personal computers and database servers continue to decline. Data warehouses that integrate clinical and financial details from patient care have become affordable, and amazing in their capacity to store and manipulate data. Users can find associations in the data that they never could have found considering the data in paper records or by using reporting functions of inflexible departmental transactions systems.

The modern decision support system environment is one designed to integrate data about patients from various specialized departmental transaction systems and to make those data available for analysis using powerful software on personal computers, communicating with the database server over a corporate network. A number of data warehouses have been created by venturesome health care organizations.[32] Many more health care organizations have acquired decision support systems from established vendors.[33] A major national conference in 1998[34] considered the use of data warehouses in health care organizations. Presenting case studies were the University of Virginia, the United States Air Force, and Catholic Healthcare West, organizations that have developed in-house clinical data warehouses for clinical quality improvement. IDX Corporation presented a commercial data warehouse, Enterprise View, initially developed and used by Inova Health System.

Spokesmen for each organization noted that use of the data warehouse did not meet their expectations. They assumed more clinicians and managers than had done so would voluntarily learn to use the data warehouse for data analysis and predictive modeling. They noted instead that managers and clinicians with access to analytical staff support chose not to use the data warehouse themselves. Those managers and clinicians without staff support are much more likely to learn to use the data warehouse themselves. Those persons using the data warehouse tend to be younger and more likely to have used computers in the past than managers and clinicians who delegate analysis to subordinates.

Most managers and clinicians express belief in the cost-effectiveness of the data warehouse but admit to insufficient skills in data analysis and personal computer software to use the data warehouse themselves. The staff of the massive data warehouse for the military health care system—CEIS (Corporate Executive Information System)[35]—tell a similar story. They have told this author that a large-scale educational program will begin in late 1998 to introduce the

*Introduction* xiii

data warehouse and tools to mine its data to personnel in the Department of Defense and in military treatment facilities worldwide.[36] Senior officers use analysts to obtain the data they need. Junior officers, except analysts, do not yet have access to the data warehouse.

Most proponents of data warehousing and hands-on analysis of data by managers and clinicians know how to use analytical software on personal computers and understand the design and purposes of relational databases. To them the benefits of corporate data available to health care leaders are obvious. They argue that today managers use their own personal computers to process their own words into electronic mail and documents. They would not have done so 10 years ago when word processing systems resided on minicomputers and users needed to know arcane commands to control the software. Then, word processors were specialists who took dictation from tape recorders and typed the words spoken into words on paper. Now personal computers and word processing software give managers a simple interface to type, or to speak, their words into print. The same transition is beginning in data analysis.

Ten years ago, the leading software for decision support—SAS, SPSS, Minitab—ran on minicomputers with arcane commands known only to a few specialists in data analysis. Now, software for data analysis on personal computers has a much more intuitive interface, handles huge data sets, and enables managers and clinicians with little skill in personal computers to interrogate their own data. The software and the hardware are not the limiting features. The ability to formulate questions for the database, and to interpret the results, are larger impediments to the usefulness of the data warehouse and the analytical tools. In other words, people need skills to work with a corporate data warehouse. They need eagerness to plumb its details and find variation in care. They need no fear of the analytical tools, the database, the data it contains, or the opportunities for quality improvement they may find in it.

Health care systems recognize that payers and patients demand:

- Lower costs.
- Demonstrated value.
- Higher quality.

The leaders of one health care system have determined that they will guide their firms' care management programs by these "fundamental principles:"[37]

1. Consistency with the values of the health care system, including commitment to optimal care of patients and to promotion of healthier communities.
2. Customer focus, both internally and externally.
3. Scientific rigor and scientific medicine.
4. Tight integration with day-to-day clinical activities.
5. Practical and pragmatic focus.
6. Focus on measurable improvements.
7. Focus on early prevention, detection, and intervention.

8. Focus on assisting integration and coordination of care delivery across patient populations, the health care continuum, and time.
9. Focus on serving the entire system, not single competing constituencies.
10. Flexible design and function to meet changing organizational and market needs.
11. Ability to demonstrate its own value.

Of the 11 fundamental principles recorded above, numbers 3, 5, 6, 8, and 11 will require of health care system leaders a thorough understanding of applied informatics if they are to accomplish the goals of their care management program. Quoting from other care management program documents[37]:

"The care management program will serve as a vehicle for sustaining and continuously improving clinical effectiveness at all RMO (regional medical organization) sites. Given the moderate degree of variability among the RMO's regions with respect to capability and needs, it is reasonable to anticipate that various programs will be piloted at one or two sites before being rolled out throughout all regions.

"For inpatient, outpatient, and preventive care, the care management program's scientific approach should feature:

- Scientific prioritization of opportunities to enhance clinical effectiveness (opportunity analysis).
- Scientific approach to best practices (benchmarking based on the medical literature).
- Scientific approach to changing provider behavior (academic detailing, opinion leaders, etc.).

"For inpatient services, the care management teams will perform these functions:

- Developmental support for scientific guidelines, pathways, and algorithms.
- Monitoring and reporting compliance with clinical practice guidelines, pathways, and algorithms.
- Analysis of current clinical practice and benchmarking.
- Performing (or assisting practitioners in performing) the core activities of scientific medicine.
- Technology assessment, as appropriate.
- Comprehensive evaluation of current or potential programs (e.g., hospitalist program), as well as:
    — Supplemental data collection.
    — Education of providers and administration.
    — Communication between departments.

# Introduction

- — Internal consulting and facilitation.
- — Provision of feedback on clinical effectiveness to customers (e.g., departments, staff, patients, payers).
- — Information and knowledge resource for customers.
- — Assisting with external activities:
  - Partnership development with purchasers and payers.
  - Response to RFPs from purchasers and payers or funding organizations focusing on clinical effectiveness.
  - Accreditation support (e.g., JCAHO, NCQA, HEDIS).
- ■ Applied clinical research

"Outside the acute care setting, the Care Management Team assumes many functions related to development support for programs in:

- ■ Demand management.
- ■ Call center.
- ■ Telemedicine.
- ■ Community education.
- ■ Self-care.
- ■ Patient education.
- ■ Care coordination across the continuum.
- ■ Ambulatory clinical guidelines.
- ■ Home care.
- ■ Disease management.

"To perform these functions, care management program staff will have these core competencies:

- ■ The ability to transform financial and clinical data into integrated information.
- ■ Clinical epidemiology and biostatistics.
- ■ Scientific medicine expertise.
- ■ Process measurement.
- ■ Outcomes measurement.
- ■ Implementation expertise, including provider and patient education.
- ■ Communication/coordination with other organizational functions.
- ■ Applied clinical research/health services research.
- ■ Process and structures to support continuous improvement.

- Decision support capability (e.g., analysis and prioritization of proposed/new programs).

"The data (simple observations with no trend analysis) and information (trended or summarized information by descriptive statistics—mean, standard deviation, range) on which the leaders and the staff of the care management program will rely include:

- Patient demographics (age, payer, sex, risk factors, etc).
- Outcomes (readmission rates, changes in quality of life, charges, costs, satisfaction, functional status).
- Clinical process data (treating physicians, follow-up home care visits, use of ACE inhibitors, education on diet).
- Clinical utilization data (levels of care, drug selection and dosing, number of cardiac or OB ECHOs obtained, length of stay).
- Operational process data (delays to specialized tests, delays in transfer to transitional or outpatient care).
- Clinical data (ejection fraction, changes in body weight, complications and comorbidity, New York Hospital Association classification)."[37]

Those data will supply an integrated patient information/knowledge base—a data warehouse. The Insight system of Catholic Healthcare West meets the criteria for a data warehouse to be used for risk adjustment (patient segmentation or stratification), treatment variation and impact, guideline development, process improvement studies, and decision support.

Without a shared, centralized data warehouse fed from clinical and financial information systems from the regional health care organizations, benchmarking of clinical processes is difficult and requires expensive manual chart review. An enterprisewide clinical and financial data warehouse is a far better alternative in support of clinical process improvement than manual chart review.

The American College of Preventive Medicine[38] and the American College of Physician Executives[39] have both developed thorough curricula for leaders of medical management programs. They have developed "competency-based education" to help their members deal with managerial issues and information technologies not seen by previous generations of clinical leaders. Lane and Ross summarized competencies and performance indicators for physicians in medical management in a recent article.[40] These are some of the topics considered an important part of competency-based education for clinical leaders in medical management:

a) Medical Management Competencies

　i) Delivery of health care

　　(1) Design, manage,, and evaluate health service delivery programs to improve the-health of a defined population.

　　　(a) This reflects demonstrated ability in:

## Introduction

xvii

(i) Design, implementation, and evaluation of clinical practice guidelines, quality management/quality improvement programs, utilization management, case management, and other activities to enhance an organization's performance and reduce practice variation.

(ii) Evaluation of health service delivery through application of techniques such as process improvement, benchmarking, outcomes assessment, and clinical epidemiology.

(iii) Analysis of the impact of managed care (e.g., HMO, POS, PPO) and other health service delivery systems/reimbursement models (e.g., fee-for-service, third-party payer, managed indemnity) on the health of defined populations; patient, payer, and provider needs and behaviors; and organizational performance.

(iv) Use of systematically collected data to prioritize system problems, identify and implement best practices, continue to improve service delivery, and assure appropriate utilization of services.

(v) Evaluation of the effectiveness, medical necessity, and appropriate use of products and interventions.

(vi) Design of systems of care that meet patient needs for access and acceptability, and measurement of patient satisfaction with these systems.

(2) Financial management

(a) Apply appropriate financial and business management techniques to ensure efficient delivery of cost-effective health services.

(i) This reflects demonstrated ability in:

1. Critical interpretation of capitation and standard financial management reports and development of recommendations to enhance organizational effectiveness.

2. Use of techniques such as cost-effectiveness analysis, cost-benefit analysis, and decision analysis (including prioritization) to allocate and manage clinical and financial resources.

(3) Outcomes management

(a) Apply organizational principles to manage a health care organization or unit.

(i) This reflects demonstrated ability in:

1. Determination of management information needs and use of medical informatics, electronic health and patient care data, and management information systems.[40]

Lane and Ross conclude their article: "Population medicine skills, which are rooted in epidemiology and biostatistics, are needed to meet societal and health care organization needs. Combined with competencies in clinical and population-based medicine, the medical management competencies and performance indicators can provide a framework for developing new residency training programs in this area."[40]

How do health care systems convey competence in population-based data analysis to clinical leaders who do not have the time, the patience, or the resources to spare to train in biostatistics, epidemiology, cost-benefit and cost-effectiveness analysis, and applied informatics? Health care systems really are not interested in conveying book learning to clinical leaders. They want to imbue clinical leaders with competence in these disciplines as quickly as possible. Competence conveys more reliably through doing exercises, not through lecture. Competence, which is the basis for knowledge, comes from accomplishing tasks and learning by doing in visceral as well as intellectual ways how to solve a problem, meet a challenge, deal with a thorny issue.

Svelby[41] argues that employee competence is the principal source of corporate wealth beyond the book value of tangible assets. He and other writers identify the incremental value of a corporation, which is greater than its book value less cash assets, with intellectual capital, which is made up of human capital, structural capital, and customer capital.

- Human capital is expertise—knowing how to solve a problem or perform a task valuable to customers or to efficient and effective operation of the firm. Knowledge, or competence, comes from practice, not from lectures and book learning. One can read about performing surgery but be utterly incompetent in the operating room until one has practiced surgical techniques in the operating room, guided by mentors with considerable surgical competence themselves. One can read management books but lack competence in the executive suite until practice in many managerial situations with ever increasing responsibility gives one competence in that setting. One accumulates human capital with experience—with practice.

- Structural capital includes some of the products of knowledge that corporations produce and own, such as patents, trademarks, policies, procedures, guidelines, manuals, instructions, databases, and networks.

- Customer capital includes relations between customers and the corporation. Some software firms enjoy extraordinary loyalty from their customers, who readily upgrade to every new release of software.

So, what skills do health care executives and clinical leaders need to acquire in order to accumulate intellectual capital in medical management? What specific capabilities must they have to accomplish the learning objectives of competence-based education in medical management? They need to have enough familiarity with managed care to know what questions to ask and enough familiarity with data analysis to know how to ask them. They need to know how to use decision support software for personal computers—such as Microsoft Access and Excel, SPSS, SAS, PowerPlay, DSS Agent, and others—to analyze data in corporate databases, data marts, and data warehouses. They need to know where to go in their organizations to obtain the data they need to phrase their questions and find answers to them. They need practice working through case studies of problems they will face as medical managers. These are some of the measurable abilities medical managers need to assess and manage health care and medical services of populations of people over time:

- Formulate a query, e.g. I wonder if this drug will produce better clinical outcomes than that drug, or I wonder if this physician makes referrals to subspecialists in the manner that this other physician does.

# Introduction

- Formulate a hypothesis in the null, for testing with standard inferential statistics.
- Interpret the data model of a data warehouse.
- Identify the transaction systems from which the data in the data warehouse came.
- Use personal computer software to access the data warehouse.
- Use a corporate network to access the data warehouse.
- Use a web browser to access the World Wide Web of the Internet.
- Use search services for the WWW (indexes and search engines).
- Explain the concept of statistical significance.
- Explain the concept of risk adjustment.
- Explain the concepts of efficiency and effectiveness.
- Formulate a question for a case study.
- Explain common medical care terms and processes of care.
- Explain the steps needed to move from data to information to knowledge to predictive modeling and calculation of expected outcomes.
- Summarize the various case mix methods used to aggregate patients into homogeneous cohorts by diagnosis and procedure codes.
- Present data in graphical format using readily available software for PCs.
- Explain cost-effectiveness and cost-benefit analyses
- Enter data into a spreadsheet and calculate fields using embedded formulas
- Use a query by example interface to formulate queries in a relational database management system, such as Microsoft Access.
- Establish a budget for data marts, or a data warehouse, for your organization.
- Explain the difficulties of data standardization limiting data analysis and creation of a data warehouse for retrospective study.
- Use predictive modeling techniques (regression, neural networks) to predict the outcomes of care for patients, and calculate expected outcomes for profiling physicians' practice habits.
- Define health care outcomes in ways both measurable and quantifiable.
- Identify the process that produces a defined outcome of interest, and measure the cost of the services and the products used in that process.
- Use a spreadsheet program to calculate capitation rates for specific populations of people, knowing incidence rates for procedure codes and costs attributable to each code.

Most leaders of care management programs know how to ask important questions for managed care programs, but not how to formulate them as hypotheses to test, or how to obtain the data to answer them, or how to analyze those data once obtained using personal computers.

So, those leaders tend not to perform the analysis themselves, but delegate it to analysts. In the process, opportunities for insights are lost. The leaders of a care management program might see many opportunities for quality improvement and conceive of dozens of additional questions if they were delving in the data directly. By remaining aloof from the details and relying on subordinates to plumb the data, they miss many opportunities for serendipity to present a pattern of care worthy of their consideration. The analytical equivalent of management by walking around is surveillance for opportunities for quality improvement by periodically interrogating corporate data warehouses, testing informed hypotheses to find trends in the data that reveal opportunities for quality improvement and cost control.

## References and Footnotes

1. http://dcri.mc.duke.edu/about/

2. Moulton, J. "Database Improves Health Care." *Duke Chronicle*, February 1996 (http://www.chronicle.duke.edu/chronicle/96/02/23/01DatabaseImproves.html).

3. Nettleman, M., and others. "Predictors of Survival and the Role of Gender in Postoperative Myocardial Infarction." *American Journal of Medicine* 103(5):357-62, Nov. 1997.

4. Harris, L., and others. "Screening for Asymptomatic Deep Vein Thrombosis in Surgical Intensive Care Patients." *Journal of Vascular Surgery* 26(5):764-9, Nov. 1997.

5. Lewandowski, K., and others. "High Survival Rate in 122 ARDS Patients Managed According to a Clinical Algorithm Including Extracorporeal Membrane Oxygenation." *Intensive Care Medicine* 23(8):819-35, Aug. 1997.

6. De Sanctis, J., and others. "Prognostic Indicators in Acute Pancreatitis: CT vs. APACHE II." *Clinical Radiology* 52(11):842-8, Nov. 1997.

7. Bailey, J. *After Thought.* New York, N.Y.: Basic Books, 1997.

8. Ortiz, J., and others. "One-Year Mortality Prognosis in Heart Failure: A Neural Network Approach Based on Echocardiographic Data." *Journal of the American College of Cardiology* 26(7):1586-93, Dec. 1995.

9. Brigatti, L., and others. "Neural Networks to Identify Glaucoma With Structural and Functional Measures." *Yearbook of Medical Informatics,* 1997, pp. 432-42.

10. Pesonen, E., and others. "Comparison of Different Neural Network Algorithms in the Diagnosis of Acute Appendicitis." *International Journal of Biomedicine and Computers* 40(3):227-33, Jan. 1996.

11. *Joint Commission Perspectives*, January/February, 1996 (http://www.jcaho.org/perfmeas/oryx/oryx_frm.htm)

12. Ruffin, M. "The Future is Here." *Physician Executive* 22(11):22-8, Nov. 1996.

13. Ruffin, M. "The Importance of Data Warehouses for Physician Executives." *Physician Executive* 20(11):45-7, Nov. 1994.

14. Ruffin, M. "Standardizing Medical Data." *Physician Executive* 23(7):61-4, Sept.-Oct. 1997.

15. Senge, P. *The Fifth Discipline, the Art and Practice of the Learning Organization.* New York, N.Y.: Doubleday, 1990.

16. Stewart, T. *Intellectual Capital, The New Wealth of Organizations.* New York, N.Y.: Doubleday, 1997.

17. Edvinsson, L., and Malone, M. *Intellectual Capital, Realizing Your Company's True Value by Finding Its Hidden Brainpower.* New York, N.Y.: Harper Business, 1997.

18. Brooking, A. *Intellectual Capital, Core Asset for the Third Millennium Enterprise.* London, England: International Thomson Publishing, 1996.

19. The Skandia Group Website: http://www.skandia.se/group/com/index.htm.

20. Fins, J. "Praxis Makes Perfect?" *Hastings Center Report* 23(5):16-9, Sept.-Oct. 1993.

21. Nolan, M., and others. "Do the Benefits of Continuing Education Outweigh the Costs?" *British Journal of Nursing* 2(6):321-4, March 25-April 7, 1993.

22. Shulkin, D., and others. "Promoting Cost-Effective Physician Behavior." *Healthcare Financial Management* 47(7):48,50,52-4, July 1993.

23. Jones, S. "Quality Improvement in Hospitals: How Much Does It Reduce Healthcare Costs?" *Journal of Healthcare Quality* 17(5);11-3; quiz 13, 48, Sept.-Oct. 1995.

24. Rutz, W. "Cost-Benefit Analysis of an Educational Program for General Practitioners by the Swedish Committee for the Prevention and Treatment of Depression." *Acta Psychiatr. Scand.* 85(6):457-64, June 1992.

25. Eckert, G., and others. "Measuring and Modifying Hospital Drug Use." *Medical Journal of Australia* 154(9):587-92, May 6, 1991.

26. Porzsolt, F., and others. "Differences between Evidence-Based Medicine and Best Conventional Medicine." *Med. Klin.* 92(9):567-9, Sept. 15, 1997.

27. Hornberger, J., and others. "When to Base Clinical Policies on Observational versus Randomized Trial Data." *Annals of Internal Medicine* 127(8 Pt 2):697-703, Oct. 15, 1997.

28. Hampton, J. "Evidence-Based Medicine, Practice Variations, and Clinical Freedom." *Journal of Evaluation in Clinical Practice* 3(2):123-31, April 1997.

29. Auplish, S. "Using Clinical Audit to Promote Evidence-Based Medicine and Clinical Effectiveness—An Overview of One Health Authority's Experience." *Journal of Evaluation in Clinical Practice* 3(1):77-82, Feb. 1997.

30. O'Neill, D., and others. "Central Dimensions of Clinical Practice Evaluation: Efficiency, Appropriateness, and Effectiveness—I. *Journal of Evaluation in Clinical Practice* 2(1):13-27, Feb. 1996.

31. Miles, A., and others. "Central Dimensions of Clinical Practice Evaluation: Efficiency, Appropriateness, and Effectiveness—II. *Journal of Evaluation in Clinical Practice* 2(2):131-52, May 1996.

32. Organizations that have created data warehouses: Inova Health System, Catholic Healthcare West, the University of Virginia, and New England Medical Center.

33. Vendors of cost accounting systems predominate: Trendstar from HBOC; Transition I, II, and IV from Transition Systems, Inc.

34. "Clinical Data Warehousing, Establishing the Value Equation." The Informatics Institute, University of Maryland Campus at Shady Grove, Thursday, June 19, 1998.

35. www.ceis.doha.mil

36. Colonel Lucas Walter, USAF, MSC, personal communication.

37. Care Management Program, internal document of Catholic Healthcare West, made available by Larimore Cummins, MD, Vice President for Care Management, Catholic Healthcare West.

38. www.acpm.org

39. www.acpe.org

40. Lane, D., and Ross, V. "Defining Competencies and Performance Indicators for Physicians in Medical Management." *American Journal of Preventive Medicine* 14(3), 229-36, April 1998.

41. Svelby, K. *The New Organizational Wealth: Managing and Measuring Knowledge-Based Assets.* San Francisco, Calif.: Berrett-Koehler Publishers, 1997.

# Contents

Foreword ..................................................................................................................i
Preface ..................................................................................................................iii
Introduction: Building Intellectual Capital—the Product of Digital Systems ........................v

## Section I—Brave New World

Chapter 1      Medical Informatics .................................................................................1
Chapter 2      On Being Digital .....................................................................................5
Chapter 3      Informatics Is a Career Management Requirement .....................................11
Chapter 4      Many Chief Information Officers Will Be Physician Executives ..............21
Chapter 5      The Politics of Informatics .....................................................................29
Chapter 6      All the News That's Fit For Bytes ...........................................................35
Chapter 7      Getting the Most Benefit from Information Systems Consultants..............39
Chapter 8      The Future of Computers........................................................................45
Chapter 9      The Future of Health Care Information Systems......................................53

## Section II—Expanding Horizons

Chapter 10     The Wonderful Evolution of Personal Computers......................................61
Chapter 11     Linking Elements of System ...................................................................69
Chapter 12     The World Wide Web Is Coming Soon to an Organization Near You........73
Chapter 13     Surfing the Web .....................................................................................79
Chapter 14     Intranets Advance Medical Care ..............................................................91
Chapter 15     Health Insurance Portability and Accountability Act of 1996 ..................101
Chapter 16     Information in a System-Oriented World................................................107

## Section III—New Structures for Health Care Delivery

| | | |
|---|---|---|
| Chapter 17 | The Organized Health Care System | 115 |
| Chapter 18 | Informatics for the Transition from Managed Care to Organized Care | 119 |
| Chapter 19 | Key Success Factors for Organized Care Systems | 123 |
| Chapter 20 | Managed Care Administration | 127 |
| Chapter 21 | Managed Care Information Needs: A Summary Perspective | 135 |
| Chapter 22 | Preparing for Managed Competition | 139 |
| Chapter 23 | New Governance for a New Era: Issues and Challenges for Integrating Systems | 149 |

## Section IV—Implications for Providers and Provider Organizations

| | | |
|---|---|---|
| Chapter 24 | Changes and Choices for Physicians | 157 |
| Chapter 25 | Physician Profiling | 163 |
| Chapter 26 | Informatics and Practice Guidelines | 173 |
| Chapter 27 | The Importance of Data Warehouses for Physician Executives | 181 |
| Chapter 28 | Telemedicine: Where Is Technology Taking Us? | 185 |
| Chapter 29 | Information Technology: A Way to Streamline Medical Practice | 189 |
| Chapter 30 | Information Technology: Interactive Media Enhance Medicine | 195 |
| Chapter 31 | Physician Executives Must Be Leaders in the Information Revolution | 199 |

**Epilog** .......................................................................................................201
**Glossary of Medical Informatics Terms** ..............................................203

# Section I

## Brave New World

# Chapter 1
## Medical Informatics

Medical informatics is an emerging science that studies the application of computing and communication technology to decision making for clinicians and managers. It enhances our understanding of how modern information and communication systems can affect the work health care managers accomplish. As the cost of technology for digital information management continues to decline relative to the costs of personnel, organizations will look for ways to offset the human costs of managing and conveying information with digital technologies.

**What Does It Mean to Store Information in Digital Form?**
Information can be stored in digital format in strings of ones and zeros that computers represent by the two states of a transistor—either charged or not charged, on or off. We have learned to condense millions of transistors into microprocessors as small as postage stamps, reducing the distance electrons need to move between transistors and increasing the occasions each second when electrons can flow between transistors. Those microprocessors can move 64 bits of data into and out of themselves hundreds of millions of times per second; they can process records from thousands of patients every second.

Can you imagine trying to find every medical record in your group practice or hospital in which a specific medication is mentioned? You may have to identify all patients who have received a certain medication if the medication is recalled because of a newly discovered adverse outcome. You would have to establish a team of people to wade through thousands of paper records, and the team would be certain to miss some of the relevant cases because of boredom or illegible records. You and everyone else involved in the search would rue the day the organization chose to keep pharmaceutical information on patients in digital form only as long as they were in the hospital or in the clinic for an appointment, after which the data would be printed to paper.

The cost of storing information in digital form on magnetic or optical disk drives is remarkably low, less than a penny to store the words that would fill hundreds of pages of paper. Managers who insist the data be printed on paper are literally being penny-wise and pound-foolish. They save the modest cost of hard disk drives and squander enormous corporate resources on paper. They may not know any better, but when is ignorance a suitable defense? Should it be a valid excuse for administrators and clinicians managing budgets for information processing? What activity in medical care does not involve processing information? We managers should ask ourselves which of those activities could be performed more effectively and efficiently if the information were in digital form?

## The New Paradigm

Why is informatics relevant now? Because health care costs continue to rise, reimbursement for visits to providers continues to shrink, and more and more providers accept capitation every day, which shifts the financial risk for the costs of care to them. Providers cannot manage their revenue the way they could under fee-for-service payment arrangements. They need to find every opportunity to reduce their operating costs. Their profit margins depend on managing costs. Why do computers matter to companies in the service sector trying to manage their operating costs? Because the clerical cost of record keeping on paper far exceeds the clerical cost of record keeping and retrieval in digital format.

Recall that the first computers cost a fortune to lease, compared to the salaries of the people operating them. A popular IBM mainframe of the 1960s, the 7090, cost about $20,000 per month to lease, while the people who operated it cost between $500 and $1,500 per month in payroll expenses. The computer was expensive and the people were cheap. Computing resources were dearly expensive and used sparingly on simple clerical work, such as payroll, claims processing, and patient accounting.

Today, however, the ratio of the costs of computing and personnel has reversed. A powerful personal computer, far more robust than the 7090 of 30 years ago, costs $200 per month to lease, but the person using it has a monthly salary of $2,000 to $20,000. Now, computers are plentiful and inexpensive, and people are the expensive resource in relatively short supply. Managers trying to reduce operating costs and improve quality of care must look for ways to replace payroll expenses with computing costs. Leaders of health care organizations need to look for every opportunity to deploy networks and computers to reduce the labor costs of data collection, storage, retrieval, and analysis. Payroll costs are the largest costs to providers of care. Computing costs continue to decline relative to payroll costs in a stunning way.

Computers are becoming easier to use and much more powerful for data processing. Every day, we find more opportunities to automate information exchange that previously was based on paper records. Every day, we make data collection and retrieval easier for the people who rely on those records to make decisions at the bedside and in the boardroom. Moving information in bits now costs less money and time than moving information in atoms, and the economic advantage to digital information management increases daily as equipment prices continue to decline relative to the costs of personnel.

## Why Is Applied Informatics Relevant to Health Care Leaders?

Leaders of medical practices, departments, and organizations of all sizes in health care know that payroll consumes most operating costs. Physicians are the most expensive resources per hour of work. Their time needs leverage wherever possible. Payers continue to reduce the income per unit of service by reducing the fees they pay for the procedures performed by physicians. Hospitals earn less for hospital stays than they once did. Payroll per employee continues to grow.

One would think that promoting efficiency in information management would be important to managers. Reduce the time nurses spend completing records. Reduce the time physicians spend trying to find records and the frequency with which they repeat diagnostic studies because the results of prior examinations cannot be found. Reduce the time patients spend visiting clinical consultants and the time consultants spend finding out what other physicians have found, performed, and prescribed. Reduce variation in practice habits and clinical outcomes among equally credentialed physicians. Increase the attention given to cost-effective screening procedures for diseases that are far less expensive to treat early than they are to treat late.

## Conclusion

To say the work habits of clinicians and managers of 20 years ago were good enough then and should be good enough now misses the fact that our wherewithal to manage information digitally has improved enormously. In the past 20 years, we have invented the personal computer and the World Wide Web of the Internet. We have produced the greatest increase in information processing efficiency in human history. The rate of improvement continues to accelerate. The costs of digital information processing have plummeted and will continue to decline for the foreseeable future. The tools at our disposal to reduce administrative and clinical inefficiencies have improved beyond belief. As stewards of health care organizations, we are obligated to learn about the new tools at our disposal and to deploy them to improve the efficiency and effectiveness of our work.

And it is fulfillment of that obligation that this book is all about. It would be impossible to describe the entirety of informatics in a single volume, but my goal here at least is to show the scope and the power of medical informatics and to convince physician executives to establish a clear role in the use of informatics in their organizations.

# Chapter 2
## On Being Digital

I've just finished reading an understated gem, *Being Digital*, by Nicholas Negroponte, Professor of Media Technology and Founding Director of the Media Lab at MIT.* It is a small paperback, fewer than 250 pages, without a single arcane term or equation in it. Yet it presents the implications of our migration from analog to digital communication with humor, grace, and simple grandeur.

He sums up our conversion from analog to digital with the disarmingly simple statement that we are switching from moving atoms of information to moving bits of information, and therein lies all the difference. It takes reflection during reading to appreciate the meaning of such a simple statement. But when you appreciate what he means, you'll thank yourself for taking the time to read what he wrote. This is a great book for a long airplane flight, or a weekend retreat, if you enjoy learning about science and technology by broad brush strokes of enthusiastic prose, full of import without technical detail.

The Media Laboratory at MIT was conceived in the late 1970s by Professor Negroponte and the then President of MIT. It was completed in 1983 with funding from charitable foundations, corporations involved in multimedia communications, and private individuals. At the time, most faculty at MIT were involved in studying technologies for computer operating systems, programming languages, and disk drives. Negroponte predicts that all programming for television, radio, and cable TV; all information currently printed in newspapers, magazines, and books; all interactive entertainment in video games and personal computer software; and all personal communications by standard and cellular telephone service will convert to digital format and will merge into one digital stream that intimately incorporates the emerging personal computer as the translator and router. Producers of information programming will have many digital avenues for distribution of their products, but all of it will be in digital format and will flow through the successors to the personal computer to the user's attention. But being digital means much more than receiving the same type of information in a new, and transparent, format. It means receiving services and products hitherto impossible in the analog format. These new products and services will transform the ways in which we practice medicine and the ways in which we manage health care.

* Negroponte, N. *Being Digital*. New York, N.Y.: Knopf, 1995.

There are many differences between analog and digital communication, but two stand out in importance. Digital communication permits the recipient, or an automated agent, to edit and correct a stream of bits before considering their meaning. And digital communication fits comfortably in a smaller electromagnetic spectrum than analog signals require, meaning that senders of information can compress more information into the signals they use to convey information to customers. The consequences to us of data correction and compression on digital data flowing into our lives are not discussed in most publications about the information age. Negroponte makes them very clear. He argues that they usher in the "post-information age," defined by our ability to act on, modify, and change the information streams coming to us to make them uniquely suited to us. In the information age, we were washed by floods of mass-produced information that everyone received in the same format and at the same time. In the maturity of the information age, each of us will receive his or her own customized stream of bits.

The implications of these changes for patient care are profound. These technologies will free us from the homogenizing influence of the mass media and give us our schedules and our preferences back. When an analog television show is on, you must watch it then, or program a VCR to catch the show in analog format to watch later. The VCR is cumbersome to use, and only about two hours of programming fits on one tape. Most of us schedule our time in front of the "tube" to attend to programs we want to watch. We watch them passively, as countless social scientists have reminded us. We modify our schedules to fit the schedule of the programs.

Would it not satisfy us more if we could program our personal computers with our preferences for subject matter to watch at home, or in the office, and trust them to sift through the sports broadcasts for the sports and teams we follow, the news subjects of importance to us, the people whose lives we want to follow, the scientific subjects about which we want to learn more, and the material we consider entertaining? Think of the thousands of hours you have "wasted" in front of television watching advertisements for products you will never buy and in which you have no interest. Think of the tens of thousands of hours your children will consume in the same way, until the bit streams into our homes are digital and we use intelligent agents, in the form of personal computers, screening out what they do not want to see. Think of saving those bits you want to save by compressing and storing them on re-writeable optical disks in your computer to be viewed and interacted with at your own time, on your own schedule.

The newspaper arrives in the morning looking the same at every home and office that receives it. Most of the information does not interest us. We skip it to find the few articles that may be of interest. But, we have to scan whole sections, and all the titles, to find the few we want to read. One morning newspaper arrives daily for hundreds of thousands, or millions of individuals in a metropolitan area. Think of the wasted type and paper and effort to deliver those papers to their destinations. And less than one hundredth of one percent of the articles, advertisements, and photographs are kept for posterity because they mean something special to someone. The newspaper is the hallmark of an analog communication medium meant to take advantage of mass production, with huge printing presses and large delivery trucks and mass marketing of the same information for everyone who receives it.

Think of all the magazines you receive with articles you don't want to read, and advertisements of no interest to you. By your subscription fees, and the prices you pay for the products and services advertised, you pay for the production and distribution of all the content that is not of interest to you. Think of the tens of thousands of articles published in medical journals every month. Most of us receive several, perhaps as many as 10, professional journals a month. Until our children are grown, we may be lucky to read one fifth of the articles in them. We may scan the index of each issue but have time to read relatively little, because we have to schedule ourselves to watch the evening news, or a sports event, when the broadcaster sends it. And we sit there wasting 20-30 percent of the time scheduled for the programming we want to watch consuming advertising of little interest to us. On the other hand, if I am considering the purchase of an automobile I might want to watch several hours of focused advertising on automobiles. But the automobile manufacturers have no way of identifying me with that sort of interest, so they must broadcast the same 30 seconds of simplistic advertising to everyone, wasting the time of most everyone watching.

Would not it be better if physician executives had an automated agent programmed by the National Library of Medicine to operate searches of the literature retrospectively, sifting through incoming professional literature for materials of particular interest to us every month and producing for us our own listings of articles most likely to be of interest? Wouldn't it be better to call up on a home computer detailed engineering content of the latest automobiles when we are ready to purchase an automobile?

Our society is just beginning to convert from analog to digital distribution of public information to home and office. I say public because private information of corporations is almost entirely digital and is distributed between computers by local and wide area networks. But those are data on customers, sales figures, and production numbers. Annual reports are still mailed in an analog brochure to every shareholder. Company newspapers and magazines still are mass produced and distributed to employees by analog mail (via interoffice mail or the postman). When we travel, our itinerary and reservations are held in digital format by airlines and hotels, but we read standard analog airline magazines and hotel visitor guides that are developed and printed with the average traveler in mind, not for you as an individual. In an analog world, mass production reduces the costs of producing each individual unit. In the digital world, we can influence the streams of bits coming at us to select what we want to know about. Merchants, including airlines and hotels, can create digital portraits of us, our preferences and tastes, to deliver to us the products and services we most value.

What does it really mean for information to be digital? On one level, it simply means that the words, or numbers, or images (moving or still), or sounds that once were stored on paper, or on film, or on tape now are stored as streams of bits on magnetic or optical disk drives and are moved from place to place as streams of electrons or photons. But that observation misses two points. Information is stored electronically, in a weightless state, and can be moved anywhere in the world in seconds with very low incremental cost, instead of on relatively heavy paper that can only be moved with considerable effort, in trucks. It means the sender can afford to customize the packaging of information for individuals at far less cost than he or she would have to pay to customize the packaging of printed information, and the recipient can act on the incoming information to select only those subjects, programs, and topics of interest and to store them electronically for consumption at leisure.

What does this conversion from atoms of information to bits of information mean to clinicians, physician executives, and patients? Everything. The same opportunities to customize the timing and content of digital information apply for individual patients, their family members, and their physicians. Instead of managing care actuarially, where the unique characteristics of all patients are averaged into homogeneous age and sex cohorts and their costs of care are predicted en masse, we will be able to manage their care epidemiologically, with specific data on each patient gathered from health risk assessments, functional status surveys, and claims data, to predict accurately the likely ailments patients will suffer and their costs of care.

With accurate information on individuals, we will practice prospective medicine. Clinicians will work with individual patients to reduce their likelihood of suffering accidents and the occurrence, or recurrence, of acute or chronic illness. The concept of prospective medicine was first promoted more than 30 years ago, but digital data on individuals, and the personal computers to manipulate those data, have become available only recently. This development will break the influence insurers have over providers. Insurers keep data sets of claims but attempt to manage the care of populations in the old way, with gross actuarial predictions by large subpopulations.

Health care providers should welcome the dawning of the era when they can manage the health of populations far more precisely. Imagine customizing each person's health care before his or her health deteriorates and he or she appears in an emergency department. The key to that transition to prospective medicine is the migration of the information about specific patients now stored in atoms of medical records to electrons of computer-based patient records. Those electrons will permit providers to manage care more precisely, predicting the likelihood of bad outcomes and intervening to prevent them from occurring.

Insurers do not have access to the medical record and cannot manage care epidemiologically. They can assemble summary medical records from claims, but they do not have clinicians' findings from histories and physical examinations, or from laboratory and radiology studies, to give them insights into the real conditions of patients. Providers can take back much of the control of their patients, which they feel they have lost to insurers, by investing in organized delivery systems that they control, and by investing in electronic information processing systems to produce computer-based patient records. Computers can interact with those electrons to give physicians clinical management possibilities they never had before. They can prescribe patient-specific health promotion information, periodic risk screenings, diet and exercise training, advice about medications, to help patients take better care of themselves.

With medical records stored in electrons, manipulated by powerful computers, moved from place to place effortlessly by electronic telecommunication networks, and stored in large databases designed for retrospective health services and clinical research, physicians will have tools with which to measure the processes of care and outcomes of their patients, including the costs of their care, and tools to gauge the practice habits of their peers. Manufacturers learned long ago that they needed to move the data in inventory, assembly, and warranty records into electrons and analyze those data by computers to identify the suppliers of parts representing the greatest warranty costs for them. Armed with specific data, they could approach suppliers and insist they improve their parts or face losing the opportunity to supply those parts.

Health care organizations need to learn the same lesson. Data and information stored in the atoms of paper do little good to the organization after the transactions they record have passed. They do not provide a ready resource for later retrospective analysis seeking opportunities for quality improvement and cost control. They do not give up their secrets easily without expensive manual chart review. Clinicians in any given specialty rarely know how other physicians in their specialty practice, because they do not refer to physicians of the same specialty. Unless they cross-cover for one another, they do not see one another's patients. Yet clinical departments of physicians are expected to develop practice guidelines together and to work systematically to improve clinical care among themselves. This is wishful thinking, at best, until physicians are in the same economic unit; a group practice or capitated physician organization of some sort; no longer face each other as courteous competitors; and share clinical details electronically.

Beyond the politics of medical care is the huge obstacle to continuous quality improvement represented by data about patients stored in atoms of paper. The discharge abstract for inpatients is available electronically, but it only includes diagnoses and procedures provided for patients. None of the findings of clinicians from histories, physical examinations, and laboratory studies that explain their decisions for treatments are in the discharge abstract. Nor are specific treatments included in the discharge abstract. The medical record needs to be stored in electrons so that studies of the characteristics of patients and the clinical decisions of physicians can be made relatively easily, by database analysis with statistics software.

When we think of computer-based records, we tend to think of computer terminals where clinicians chart their notes, enter their orders, or look up results, as if the medical record were pasted on the computer screen the way text and numbers about patients are attached to paper. We may think of the computer keyboard with trepidation, or loathing, because it is harder for most of us to use than pen and paper. Intuitively, we know how to thumb through paper. Do not think of the computer as a substitute for paper. If you do, you will ignore services and functions electronic documents give us, and additional actions we can take with computer-based patient records that empower clinicians to deliver much better clinical care than they ever could without the benefit of electronic clinical records. When you transform the information about patients from atoms to bits, opportunities to enhance health and medical care flourish.

# Chapter 3
## Informatics Is a Career Management Requirement

Executives in every industry need to understand how promising new technologies will affect their businesses, but especially those in industries where rapid information processing is vital to success. For executives in health care, the evolving marketplace for managed care makes efficient information processing and telecommunications indispensable to manage effectively a single physician's practice or a large multinational conglomerate. Unfortunately, most managers have grown up without learning to use personal computers and are just starting to read about technological innovations, such as the Internet's World Wide Web, that will have profound influences on their work and lives. Physician executives need to understand applied informatics in order to lead their organizations wisely and successfully into major investments in standardized electronic records, telecommunication networks, multimedia workstations, and new services, such as telemedicine.

Just as clinicians must learn to use superior diagnostic and therapeutic technologies as they become available, such as antibiotics, anesthesia, electrocautery, insulin, chemotherapy, linear accelerators, and magnetic resonance imaging, so, too, must physician executives learn about standardized clinical lexicons and computer-based patient records, relational databases, data repositories for retrospective data analysis, telecommunication technologies, and the Internet. They also need to learn about computer-based patient records, outcomes management, practice guidelines, expert systems for differential diagnosis, knowledge bases and electronic medical textbooks on the Internet, and community health information networks (CHINs). The latter can be used to inform patients about how to manage chronic conditions, learn to take better care of themselves, prepare for diagnostic studies and surgical procedures, and schedule preventive health measures.

The most substantial investments health care organizations make in the next decade will be in electronic data and information processing systems to support efficient and effective delivery of clinical services. To lead their organizations, physician executives will need to understand the functions and limitations of these systems. Knowledge is power. Managing the myriad health care services needed for defined populations of people over time, under fixed budgets set by capitation, requires timely, accurate, and standardized information processing and sharing among all providers involved. You can't manage what you can't measure.

Physician executives manage the clinicians caring for those populations. Increasingly, they are asked to participate in procuring the information systems needed to expedite data collection, sharing, and analysis. A patient's paper medical record in a specific setting must be supplanted by a health record available electronically to all clinicians treating that individual, regardless of their locations within the health care delivery system.

Physician executives study marketing, finance, health law, and organizational behavior, even though they will usually delegate specific duties related to those areas. In the same way, physician executives need to know what technological trends, threats, and opportunities their directors of information systems face, even though they may not aspire to direct those departments themselves. Imagine the chief executive of a bank who does not spend considerable time studying how to obtain and deploy the best information processing technologies. Try to imagine a segment of our economy that is more information intensive, and more information dependent, than the health care industry.

## An Applied Science

Informatics involves the application of information systems and the processes for selecting, installing, and operating the systems. It does not address theories of software, hardware, or firmware. It explores technological trends that will affect the types of information processing systems available. It does not look at the physics and mathematics of technologies that are not feasible, yet. Informatics is practical and applied. It is not about breakthroughs in electrical engineering or about the likely design of future systems. It is about the technologies applicable to the business of health insurance and providers today.

Informatics helps clinicians, leaders, and managers learn to use information processing and communication technologies in much the same way that one learns to drive an automobile. We learn that there are common rules of the road—national standards for parking, turning, traffic signals. People can drive any car, anywhere in the United States and in most foreign countries, as long as they adhere to the basic rules of driving (steering wheel on the left, driving on the right side of the road). In much the same fashion, informatics teaches standards for data collection, storage, retrieval, communication, and analysis that permit health care organizations everywhere to use electronic medical records and data repositories for retrospective analysis, quality control, and outcomes assessment.

## Widely Available

The worldwide personal computer industry, including hardware, software, and related services, represents more than $150 billion per year in sales. Most who invest in computer technology are not technophiles squandering money on new toys, or neophytes duped by proselytizing vendors. Most are people who perform useful work with those technologies, producing more benefits than the cost of the initial investment.

Computers of all sizes, including advanced calculators, can be found in all but the very smallest businesses. School children reach their teens knowing how to use personal computers. Executives learn to type their own letters and produce their own budgets on PCs because their companies can no longer afford secretaries for each of them. E-mail is an indispensable asset.

# Informatics Is a Career Management Requirement

More than 20,000 e-mail messages per second move over the Internet during working hours, and that number is rising rapidly with growing use of the Internet.

Many professional schools and undergraduate programs require students to have computers. Students obtain their syllabi, class notes, and exercises over school networks and climb onto the Internet to access information from government agencies, libraries, commercial ventures, and other students for homework and research projects. When they graduate into the work force, they will use those same skills to find data and information for research reports, marketing studies and business plans.

Nurses and physicians completing training have learned to use computer-based patient record systems to enter orders and retrieve laboratory results, at least for inpatients. Most organizations offering training programs for physicians and nurse practitioners who specialize in primary care plan to install computer-based patient records in their clinics. The new generation of clinicians knows how to use computers, and expects to use them in their practices. The personal computer and electronic networks are essential enabling technologies.

## Endogenous Growth

In the 1950s, economists argued that humans would overpopulate the world and starve, unable to make sufficient food. We have discovered that we can produce more food now than was ever dreamed of 40 years ago. We have developed communication and information processing technologies unimaginable then. We have created a biotechnology revolution and the promise of better treatments for disease. People submit more patent applications every year.

Many devices and methods for minimally invasive, endoscopic surgery have been developed to reduce trauma. Physicians have learned to change their practice habits and to reduce their dependence on hospitals as new medications, procedures, and treatments allow expanded outpatient care. Health care organizations find ways of using the Internet to influence the unhealthy habits of patients. The principal resource in the quest for continuous improvement is patient data studied for signs of outcome variation. We need to build learning organizations, as Peter Senge, author of *The Fifth Discipline*,[1] says, and this requires observational data analysis to identify better ways of performing the processes of management and care.

We dream of achieving what we previously thought impossible and then figure out how to attain it. The ideas we need to continue to improve health care will emerge from clinical and health services research. Applied informatics will help us identify, standardize, collect, and analyze data about our patients and health plan members to reveal opportunities for quality improvement.

## Who Needs to Learn Informatics?

Most leaders of health care organizations—health plans, hospitals, group practices, insurance companies, pharmaceutical firms, and suppliers to the industry—have not used computers. They finished their formal education before personal computers were useful and generally do not become involved in planning to computerize information systems. They approve the budgets, once they are reassured that these systems will save money for their organization over five years, but they don't participate in system implementation. Computer systems are used to automate specific clerical tasks and not the stuff of corporate strategy, or so they think.

With widespread consolidation of payers and providers and the advent of regionally integrated delivery systems, and with providers taking financial risk for the care of populations, computer-based patient records will be any health care organization's key asset. Informatics will be one of the most important disciplines for them to understand if health care leaders are to help their organizations use these expensive and transforming technologies successfully. Right now, regional group practices of physicians are forming, many funded by hospitals and physicians, some by physicians and venture capitalists. Their first major investments are in standardized office practice systems and networks linking the locations where they practice to create and share computer-based patient records.

**Direct User Access to Computers**
Thousands of years ago, scribes wrote down whatever their leaders wanted them to commit to papyrus. Until 600 years ago, books were copied by hand. When Thomas Jefferson attended college, many students employed secretaries to take notes. As tools have made production less expensive, most people have learned to create their own documents. Not only do students take their own lecture notes, but employees from all kinds of enterprises, including senior managers, produce documents on computers. Secretaries rarely take dictation anymore—their bosses type memos and letters, send e-mail, and draft reports on their PCs. Most physicians still scrawl short progress notes for office and hospital visits and dictate other clinical reports. Speaker-independent voice recognition systems will make the intermediary far less common.

Imagine you run a hospital. All else being equal, you would prefer physicians who can retrieve patient laboratory results from the computer than ones who depend on nurses to get information for them. Imagine you are in charge of a corporation, and you have a choice of a manager who can use a personal computers and one who depends on staff to do the same work. All else being equal, would you prefer the one who can collect data and create documents, especially if he or she produces the work faster and at a lower clerical cost? Investing in computer technologies to help employees obtain and use information quickly, and training them to do so, define the purpose of applied informatics.

**How Will Others Use These Informatics Tools?**
Managers approve budgets for information and communications systems that amount to tens of thousands of dollars in hardware, software, and consulting for small group practices, hundreds of thousands of dollars for group practices of 30 to 100 physicians, millions of dollars for single hospitals and health plans, and tens of millions of dollars for multihospital systems. Traditional administrators are trained to manage facilities. Most of them are not familiar with the uses of telecommunication networks, clinical decision support systems, and computer-based patient records. But their organizations will pour as much money into computer systems in the next 10 years as they put into facilities in the past 10 years. Those managers need training in informatics to understand and successfully manage these investments.

**Computer-Based Patient Records: The Most Important Asset**
Computer-based patient records (CPRs) will be the most important resource for managing the care of populations of patients and health plan members. They can be used to enhance patient satisfaction, while controlling spending and standardizing and improving the quality of care delivered. CPRs for hospitals, health plans, and physician networks are not software packages from single vendors. In larger health care organizations, the CPR is made up of a standardized data dictionary and data models on which all users agree, multimedia workstations

to collect data, relational data repositories to store data, networks to communicate data, and separate relational databases for retrospective analysis of data. The databases, standardized data elements, workstations, and networks must be integrated into one shared computer architecture if the organization is to avoid squandering financial resources on software and systems that are incompatible, redundant, or otherwise useless.

## Windows to the Digital World

Executives need to learn about informatics to know how to access the Internet's World Wide Web and find information key to their work and organizations. The Web's growth rate is faster than for any other man-made product in history. A new home page is added every four seconds. The number of users doubles every two months. Disks arrive in the mail from a wide range of companies offering inexpensive access for effortlessly loading their software. And the number of such access routes continues to grow exponentially.

Those already on the Web can download new versions of Netscape and Microsoft Internet Explorer for free and enjoy multimedia features. The number of servers with interesting documents available to Web browsers grows exponentially, attracting new users every minute. The Web is the precursor of the information superhighway, with all its multimedia offerings.

The speed of modems is not increasing as rapidly—it has risen more than eightfold, from 300 baud (bits per second) to 57,600 baud in the past 12 years—but interest in the Web encourages telecommunication companies to invest in and develop faster digital access, with communication protocols such as ISDN ( about $30-40 per month in urban areas), switched 56 kilobit (56,000 bits per second) dedicated lines, cable modems, and faster digital line signaling protocols that promise to carry data at millions of bits per second over the standard twisted pair copper wires we already use for telephone calls.

What was impossible only a few years ago is possible today. Our habits of thinking change much more slowly than our technology. We find ourselves required to use a mouse—a toy used by our children yesterday—much sooner than we expected. Today they are attached to the computers in our group practices and hospitals, and we must use them to obtain patients' laboratory results to care for them promptly.

## Can Managers Avoid Technology?

Can senior executives avoid the responsibility of using personal computers to access corporate data; read and produce e-mail; and create memos, letters, and reports? When is an executive so important that the organization will let him or her not use a personal computer that provides access to vital corporate data faster, and at lower expense, than asking staff to get those data? When is a hospital or group practice likely to require that all clinicians enter data into computer-based patient records?

What do we do with the executive who cannot retrieve information from the corporate network? What do we do with the executive who cannot produce a letter? What do we do with the hospital or group practice executive who must approve a multimillion dollar budget for computer-based patient records but has no notion of what a computer-based patient record looks like, how clinicians can use it to improve patient care, or what training is required to use the CPR to full advantage?

Managers and clinicians who think they are too old, or too important, to learn to use a personal computer need to think again. We ought not to tolerate the manager or clinician who refuses to use e-mail, because in many circumstances it is the most efficient means of leaving a message. E-mail will be replaced by multimedia mail and video conferencing that will be based on the Web and will be less expensive than long-distance telephone calls. In fact, long-distance telephone calls will change to Internet calls. Vinton Cerf, a Senior Vice President of MCI and one of the developers of the Internet, recently summed up the growth of the Internet with a few statistics. At the beginning of 1998, there were approximately 40 million regular users of the Internet, with their numbers growing by 1,000,000 each month. From January 1996 through January 1997, the traffic in packets over the portion of the Internet backbone managed by MCI (now MCI Worldcom) grew 15% per month. MCI anticipates a growth rate of 300% per year in the demand for digital bandwidth for Internet traffic. MCI assumes the numbers of packets per second devoted to the Internet will grow by a factor of nine every two years, and by 729 every six years. Voice traffic is growing slowly over MCI circuits, about 5 percent per year. By the year 2000, data traffic over the MCI network will surpass voice traffic. MCI Worldcom will cease to be a voice telephone company, becoming a local and wide-area communications company for all forms of digital communication—voice, data, video, still images.[2]

Clinicians who avoid learning to use workstations for video conferencing will miss opportunities to communicate with their patients in their homes, to take medical care to the patient, and to make more informed triage decisions. They will miss the chance to place documents now printed and distributed by mail—schedules of health education events, policy and procedure manuals, newsletters, directions to treatment facilities, and explanations of diagnoses and treatments in layman's terms—on the Web, making them available to the community at a lower cost.

How does a physician-hospital organization, management services organization, or group practice that is acquiring physicians' practices value a group practice in which the physicians have not automated any processing of documents, with all scheduling, accounting, and medical records based on paper forms? Would the potential acquirer avoid practices that have not organized and standardized their records electronically? What are the risk management issues for physicians' practices that do not use decision support software to help clinicians select medications and determine dosages, identify potential drug-drug interactions, avoid allergic reactions, reduce adverse reactions due to disordered physiological parameters in patients, or formulate differential diagnoses in complex cases?

What do we do with academic physicians who cannot obtain literature from the National Library of Medicine's Medline? Do we insist that they learn to use Grateful Med via the Internet, PaperChase, or other online knowledge bases? Physicians who cannot look up articles on how to manage patients with complex cases may not practice medicine as successfully as those who do. The latter may gain insight into best practices faster than their less technologically savvy colleagues.

Physicians and managers who cannot enter data into computers about patient treatments and outcomes may not discern patterns that could lead to new and better case management ideas. Without systematic study, it is unlikely that those managers or physicians will see opportunities for quality improvement. A learning organization expects its members to look for ideas that improve its work processes. It creates good outcomes for its customers by successful implementation and continuous improvement of care processes.

What does the learning organization do with the clinician who does not use patient education software to print instructions about clinical conditions and treatments? Standardized instructions can answer questions patients don't ask during office visits and reduce the likelihood of unnecessary resource consumption. The more informed patients are about their ailments, the better they follow instructions and manage symptoms, with less dependence on the health care system. A lack of effort in patient education may well cost the health care system more resources in the long run.

What happens to physicians who lose contracts because payers want to work only with those who use computer-based patient records? If an IPA, PHO, or multispecialty group practice adopts a computer-based patient record, physicians who wish to participate fully in patient care will implement and use that system. Physicians in a group practice or hospital are expected to complete their clinical records on paper forms standardized by the facility in which they work. As hospitals and group practices adopt electronic medical records, they will expect physicians to use them.

Physicians and hospitals who need to store paper records (storage space costs $10 to $25 per square foot) could save money by using electronic medical records and putting them on "write once read many" (WORM) drives, a technology for recording data on optical media in such a way that they cannot be edited or overwritten but can be read multiple times. When providers feel the squeeze of diminishing premiums and capitation rates, the storage space dedicated to paper records will become more of an issue.

Physicians and hospitals are beginning to create and use pages on the Web. Already, in major metropolitan areas, a substantial segment of the population explores the Web. People will become accustomed to learning about and purchasing products and services over this medium. Hospitals and physician groups that use the Web to inform members of the public about their services and the ways they can participate in managing their care will find market share shifting their way. Passwords and encryption can protect the privacy of those using the Web.

Patients and plan members will abandon providers who do not have electronic communication. When many physicians accept e-mail from patients, those who do not will lose patients. When hospitals allow patients scheduled for elective procedures to preregister electronically from home so they do not have to complete forms while waiting in the admissions department, those that do not offer this service will miss the boat.

Health care systems with relatively high operating expenses will lose patients to those that cost less, especially if they cannot prove that they provide higher quality services or better outcomes. Informatics is needed to measure quality and value and to reduce operating costs. The techniques involve data collection about patient outcomes (mortality, charges, functional status, and satisfaction), storage of standardized data in a relational database, and systematic analysis of those data to find opportunities for quality improvement and reduction of outcome variations. Organizations that invest in relational database management systems for storage of data on patient care processes are more likely to find ways to reduce costs and improve outcomes, making themselves more attractive to purchasers of health care services.

To the winners of the cost and quality wars will go the spoils of more patients and more health plan members.

Many states require that health plans receive accreditation by the NCQA to maintain licensure. Health plans need to report process and outcome data, based on the Health Plan Employer Data and Information Set (HEDIS) statistics. If their current providers cannot provide such data, payers will have no recourse but to contract with those who do. For instance, Aetna-U.S. Healthcare demands that physicians and hospitals submit data for HEDIS reports in a timely manner. If they don't, they receive smaller payments and smaller bonuses.

## Refining Risk Adjustments

What happens to organizations that can't risk-adjust clinical data to be used for physician profiling, outcomes studies, and quality improvement programs? They misinterpret patient outcomes, alienate physicians who know what analyses are needed, and lose the opportunity to interest medical staffs in quality improvement.

Clinicians understand that every patient is different and that patients arrive for care with specific probabilities for each health outcome that is possible. Obese, hypertensive, hypercholesterolemic, inactive diabetic patients who smoke cigarettes are far more likely to suffer illnesses that require medical intervention than svelte patients with none of those bad health habits, no matter what their physicians do for them. The physician burdened with more of the former patients will be associated with a higher frequency of negative outcomes than the physician who doesn't treat them—intentionally or unintentionally.

Consider two physicians who treat patients with cancer. One can show that his patients have a 93 percent chance of living five years after initial treatment for their malignancies. The other shows with equally valid outcomes data that patients have a 7 percent chance of living five years after treatment. Who is the better physician? Of course, you need to know if they treat patients with the same kind of cancer. You understand that patients arrive with differing probabilities of a certain outcome depending on their underlying condition. In this example, the physician with the large proportion of patients surviving five years is a dermatologist treating basal cell carcinomas of the skin. The second is an oncological surgeon treating patients with carcinoma of the pancreas. Because the patients differ in the types of cancer they suffer, their probabilities of death within five years after treatment vary.

What education, training, and informatics technologies are organizations acquiring to refine risk adjustment where the prior probabilities of common outcomes—mortality, cost, wound infection, functional status, and satisfaction—vary by patient? Managers need to be involved in decisions about education, training, and information technology, because they determine the basic budgets for information systems, health services research, and all other investment and operating expenses for their organizations.

## The Web

The Internet, specifically the World Wide Web, will transform computing and electronic communication with standards for multimedia information exchange. Most Westerners know the Web as a network to send and receive e-mail and colorful documents. Most people do not realize, yet, that the Web is designed for multimedia communication between computers, including data entry and retrieval with sounds, images, video, and graphics as well as text.

Bandwidth, the speed at which data files move from computer to computer, is still a limitation, but, as people discover the Web's capabilities, they will invest in faster digital access. Around the corner, but available before the year 2000, is technology to move millions of bits per second over standard copper telephone lines. The Web is the application that will urge us to faster digital access and give us a vehicle for efficient and pleasant electronic and digital voice, text, image, and video communication.

The desire to move quickly and to communicate makes these investments inevitable. We will think nothing of paying $25 to $75 per month for fast digital communication. We'll get basic telephone and cable television service, access to the Web, and the ability to videoconference for less than we pay for telephone, cable television, cellular telephone, and online access today. Vendors of application programs, including word processors, online encyclopedias, and home banking/finance systems, will adopt graphical user interfaces that seamlessly integrate with Web browser software for access to information and entertainment without having to move between programs.

The rush to Web standards for sharing data will advance vendors' commitment to making computer-based patient records, patient education applications, and office practice management systems. This will not be hard, because most have adopted the Microsoft Windows® interface. The Internet will already be embedded in these companies' software, making the job of moving patient data reliably and securely easier than it is now using incompatible, proprietary systems.

But what happens to the physician's office, health plan, or hospital that doesn't adopt this new, open, and shared standard for clinical computing? Will they receive patients' information electronically? No, they won't—or, if they do, it will be at a high price. Will they send data to other organizations involved in patient care quickly and reliably? Not without expensive, proprietary interfaces.

You've probably selected a bank with a debit card that you can use at most automatic teller machines, because it uses standard and popular financial networks such as MOST, Cirrus, and others. The same dynamics will happen in health care. As clinical networks emerge using Internet standards, those that link physicians to only one hospital or payer will lose favor quickly. Organizations will need to move to standardized networks that allow secure communication of multimedia data, and they will undoubtedly be based on the Web design.

**The Promise of Telemedicine?**
Telemedicine is for patients who would prefer to have a teleconference from home that answers their questions rather than drive to a physician's office, an urgent care clinic, or an emergency department? Telemedicine will expand as video teleconferencing grows on the Web. By adhering to Web standards, hospitals and physicians will be able to participate with patients in video teleconferences without having to pay for, install, or maintain proprietary equipment on patients' PCs. Woe to the organization or private medical practice that does not see this standardization coming and instead invests in systems that do not support Internet standards.

Woe, also, to the provider organization that does not offer staff the resources to support telemedicine consultations after the public learns to expect videoconferencing for banking, shopping, and other activities. The health care organization that offers home and office health care conferences with providers will attract new business. Banks that did not offer automatic teller machines lost business to those that did—and now all offer ATMs. Travel agents who only scheduled flights on one airline lost out to those who could compare fares and schedules of all the major airlines. Grocery stores that did not use universal bar codes to tabulate customers' purchases lost to those that did.

Providers who will not submit claims electronically are paid less, or not paid at all, by large insurers. Medicare demands electronic claims submission from hospitals, and soon will for all physicians' offices. Customers will expect telemedicine, and their health plans will promote its use as a way to reduce the cost of unnecessary visits to urgent care centers and emergency departments. Physicians who receive capitation will organize telemedicine services, probably staffed by nurse practitioners and physicians' assistants, for initial triage decisions for the same reasons.

## Conclusion

Informatics is an indispensable discipline for leaders and managers because the most important assets of their organizations are their information processing technologies and because the key skills are those that help them to manage information. Managers and executives increasingly will need to anticipate trends in information management technologies that could affect their businesses. In health care, computer-based patient records, integration engines, online analytical processing systems, telemedicine, expert systems, and the Internet have become vital to a competitive advantage. Leaders who do not understand the promise and limitations of these technologies and those who do not understand the importance of strong leadership to establish standards for data and transaction systems will not lead their organizations well.

## References

1. Senge, P. *The Fifth Discipline: The Art and Practice of the Learning Organization.* New York, N.Y.: Currency/Doubleday, 1990.
2. Speech by Vinton Cerf at Infocom 1997: http://www.ckp.or.jp/infocom97.

# Chapter 4
## Many Chief Information Officers Will Be Physician Executives

In the next century, clinicians, most of whom will be physician executives, will lead the operation of, and investment in, information and communication systems for many health care organizations. And in the first decade of the next century, most health care organizations will recruit clinicians to manage those departments. Why? Because health care delivery systems will have substantial financial incentives to invest in clinically oriented information technologies to measure and manage the practices of their clinicians, to ease the burden on clinicians of collecting clinical details about patients in electronic form, to alert clinicians to practice guidelines adopted by the delivery systems in which they practice, and to increase the efficiency of data communication about patients to clinicians in their homes and offices.

Organized delivery systems, capitation payments to providers, practice guidelines, and profiling of physicians' practice habits will change the power structure in departments of information systems from one that favors financial processing for billing for procedures to clinical processing for clinical data collection, communication, and analysis to make health care services as efficient and effective as possible. If patients are to be identified electronically at all locations of care within an integrated delivery system, and if the findings of clinicians and treatment decisions are to be codified electronically for electronic storage and distribution in computer-based patient records, behind the clinical information systems must be enormous effort at standardization of clinical vocabularies and medical records. The growing importance of standardized electronic medical records will bring clinicians quite naturally to leadership positions in departments of information systems.

Many people are interested in comparing the effectiveness and efficiency of various ways of treating patients. As a society, we need to measure the relative merits of alternative ways of treating specific medical conditions. There are no direct measures of efficiency or effectiveness, because there are no standard scales for efficiency and effectiveness. The measures we use, such as costs of care, charges for care, cure rates, mortality rates, five-year survival rates, patient satisfaction scores, and patient functional status scores, all are proxies for the concepts we want to measure—efficiency and effectiveness. Increasingly important to clinicians and institutions will be comparisons of their effectiveness and efficiency to include, or exclude, them from alternative delivery systems such as HMOs, IPAs, PPOs, PHOs, and OWAs (other weird arrangements).

Profiling providers for inclusion in, or exclusion from, delivery systems already occurs. It affects subspecialists more than primary care physicians, who usually are more attractive to alternative delivery systems, and occurs more often in urban areas, where concentrations of all providers are highest. Until recently, profiling by insurers has been inclusive in nature, ruling out those few clinicians with unacceptable malpractice histories or inadequate credentials and those few facilities that do not meet the standards for accreditation of the Joint Commission on Accreditation of Healthcare Organizations. Most payers say they can no longer afford to include all providers in their networks.

In order to compare the outcomes of patients and measure the relative effectiveness and efficiency of specific treatment methods, we must control for each patient's prior probability of the outcome on which the comparisons depend. Before treatment, patients come to clinical trials with varying probabilities of the outcome of interest to researchers. Before they are treated, patients with cancer vary in their probabilities of surviving five years. Some of them suffer with cancers that are widely metastatic, while others are blessed with tumors still localized and eradicable through surgery and/or radiation therapy.

Therefore, comparing the outcomes of treatments for patients depends on fairly comparing patients' prior probabilities of the outcomes under study before treatments are introduced. This is as true for academic research designed to compare the outcomes of patients treated with alternative experimental drugs as it is when profiling physicians to compare the effectiveness and efficiency of their clinical practices. An endocrinologist who has filled his practice with svelte, young, athletic, diabetic patients whose blood sugars are controlled well with diet and exercise and who have no measurable end-organ injury from microvascular disease will measure far better outcomes for his patients, in terms of costs of care, rates of complications and hospitalization, and rates of referral to other consultants, than an endocrinologist whose patients are obese, elderly diabetics requiring complex regimens of insulin and already suffering with multiple end-organ injury. In order to compare fairly the performance of these two endocrinologists, we must control for the probabilities of specific outcomes among their patients before they began to treat them.

We can control for prior probabilities of the outcomes under study in one of two ways. Either we carefully control the patients entered into a clinical trial, to make certain that patients are comparable in all ways except for the treatments the outcomes of which are being compared, or we use statistical techniques (regression analysis) to control for variations in patients' prior probabilities of the outcomes in question.

Health care organizations need health services research staff who know how to analyze clinical data for presentation to committees wrestling with clinical quality improvement initiatives, developing clinical practice guidelines, or profiling the practice habits of clinicians. Health services research staff need to work closely with information systems staff who create the data models, data dictionaries, and databases for data analysis. Far better for them to work side by side in the same department of information systems than to sequester them in separate cost centers where they will tend to work independently, and often competitively, duplicating efforts and producing inconsistent data resources and analyses.

Departments of information systems of health care organizations usually are not at the center of clinical data collection and analysis, in part because they are usually led by managers who are not familiar with clinical practice. They usually report to vice presidents of finance. Data collection and analysis are performed throughout health care organizations, usually by staff reporting to various middle managers in charge of marketing, human resources, finance, risk management, quality improvement, quality assurance, and clinical research. These fragmented services usually do not collaborate on a standardized nomenclature for defining the findings and experiences of patients, or on risk-adjustment methods for the prior probabilities of patients' outcomes, or on standardized ways of presenting data analysis to clinicians and managers. Each department head has his or her own analytical staff. Usually they do not establish common databases for analytical work.

Health care organizations now feel the pressure to invest in data warehouses for retrospective analysis, because clinicians' and managers' interest in data collection and ad hoc analysis is growing with the increasing turbulence in the marketplace for health care services. There is increasing urgency to perform ad hoc analysis of health care data to respond promptly to requests for proposals from insurers and to demands for outcomes data from regulatory agencies and the media. In the absence of a corporate data warehouse containing all financial and clinical data on patients, small, incompatible, inconsistent databases crop up under the guidance of data analysts in the various departments mentioned above, with little or no standardization among them of data definitions, data formatting, data modeling, query design, or risk adjustment.

Information systems traditionally have not played a leading role in decision support for health care organizations. Finance and accounting have played that role, with financial information systems giving them their data. That orientation must change to support clinical quality improvement, development of practice guidelines, and standardized profiling of clinicians' practice habits. No other department is better positioned than information systems to play this crucial role of maintaining and protecting the information resources of the organization, including transaction systems, communication networks, and data repositories for retrospective analysis of clinical and financial data. Departments of information systems must take on a sales orientation and analyze the needs of their customers for useful information and communication resources before their customers ask for them. They need to go after opportunities to help clinicians and managers improve the work that they do.

The key technological trend that is moving information systems to the forefront of clinicians' attention is the rapidly increasing power of personal and mid-range computers that, with graphical user interfaces and fast microprocessors attached to corporate networks, can give clinicians windows to an electronic world of multimedia data about their patients—alphanumeric text, sounds, images, graphics, and video—from any terminal in their health care facilities, in their offices, and in their homes. Now there is no technological impediment to collecting, storing, transmitting, and displaying every component of the medical record electronically on personal computers attached to wide-area networks of regional health care organizations. The personal computer workstation becomes the clinicians' power tool for access to patients' demographic and clinical data and to databases designed for retrospective inquiry into the treatments and outcomes of many patients. Databases for decision support are becoming the principal resources for clinical quality improvement and outcomes analyses for all health care organizations.

Departments of information systems already maintain transaction systems for financial data processing. Usually, they also maintain information systems for clinical transaction processing, such as laboratory, pharmacy, and radiology systems. They manage telecommunication networks that move data from servers to workstations and back again. But departments of information systems usually do not maintain the departmental data repositories, such as tumor, transplant, and trauma registries, used for recording the clinical treatments and outcomes of patients. Usually, departments of medical records are not part of departments of information systems. Medical records departments, when they move to electronic storage of medical records in computer-based document processing systems, usually do not include departments of information systems in their planning or implementation. They hire outside consultants to help them draft requests for proposals to send to vendors recommended by the consultants or identified in exhibits at national meetings of medical records professionals. Departments of finance usually do not involve information systems in procurements for cost accounting systems. They also tend to hire outside consultants to lead them through procurements of cost accounting software and only involve departments of information systems when interfaces are required between the newly selected cost accounting systems and the existing patient accounting systems.

All of these independent decisions made by autonomous operating departments lead to a polyglot of data definitions for key clinical concepts and later to difficulty in standardizing clinical nomenclatures to define findings and treatments for patients. Not all clinical registries use ICD-9-CM codes for diagnoses and procedures. Some clinical departments, such as orthopedic surgery, need extensions of the ICD-9-CM methodology; some need nomenclatures to describe anatomic findings of patients, such as SNOMED III; some need unstandardized terms to describe clinical findings, such as measurements taken at cardiac catheterization; and some need data from their own idiosyncratic survey instruments that measure patient satisfaction and functional status.

Let me suggest a job description for a clinical chief information officer. The CIO must supervise and manage the organization that installs, implements, maintains, and upgrades electronic information and communication technologies. Usually, an administrative CIO does these things and not much more. A clinical CIO will also lead clinicians to successful data standardization, collection, and analysis for clinical quality improvement and outcomes management. The clinical CIO will create and supervise a division of clinical informatics devoted to data collection and risk adjustment to support profiling of physicians and research studies for clinical quality improvement exercises. The clinical CIO will teach clinicians and managers to understand the benefits, costs, and limitations of computer-based patient records and will lead standardization of those records, including clinical departmental data repositories, such as tumor, transplant, and trauma registries, to support patient care. The clinical CIO will lead the development of teleconferencing capabilities to support telemedicine programs to more remote populations underserved by subspecialists. The clinical CIO will lead the training of administrative and clinical staff on personal computers to permit them to perform their own retrospective data analysis using risk-adjustment methods and databases standardized for the organization.

The key to successful electronic communication is standardization—for data, for software applications, for operating systems, for hardware, for networks. In fact, standardization of computer records is much more important than standardization of paper records, because humans can recognize patterns in text and on paper of various sizes and shapes much easier than computers can. Leading the standardization of clinical and financial systems to support computer-based patient records for on-line transaction processing and retrospective analysis is perhaps the most important role of the clinical chief information officer.

You might ask why health care organizations may not be better served by having two CIOs— a layman who knows computer and communications technologies intimately and who has supervised operations of departments of information systems before as chief information officer, and a clinician as clinical information officer, reporting to the layman and leading standardization of clinical nomenclatures, selection of clinical transaction systems, and data analysis for quality improvement and guideline development. My observation is that the tone and tempo of an organization, like an orchestra, is set by the conductor. I believe the conductors of organizational informatics of large health care organizations must know clinical work intimately. If this is the case, why are there not more clinicians as CIOs? The rest of administration of a health care system may be anxious about a clinician CIO, because they have never dealt with one before. The CEO of a health care system may not want a clinical CIO, or any CIO, reporting to him because he does not feel competent to guide someone with training in technologies beyond his ken.

Such risk-averse CEOs need to go into retirement, and clinical CIOs need to report to CEOs who are not afraid to learn what they need to learn to support and guide their CIOs to create information and communication systems supporting electronic collection, storage, communication, retrieval and analysis of data on patients and operations. After all, those information systems are becoming the most important tangible assets of the emerging health care systems those CEOs are paid to lead.

Health care organizations need clinicians to lead rather than to advise administrators. The clinician CIO can be a nurse, physical or respiratory therapist, pharmacist, or physician. However, while allied health professionals with training in information systems are invaluable for selection and implementation of clinical transaction systems, such as order entry and results reporting systems, physicians will be more likely to succeed in leading other physicians to adopt and use computer-based patient records, to standardize their data collection in the office to support computer-based patient records for inpatients and outpatient use, and to collect and analyze data from clinical processes and outcomes for profiling the efficiency and effectiveness of alternative clinical treatments. The table on pages 27 and 28 lists some of the specific projects related to information and communication systems that many CIOs are wrestling with now, or will face in the near future. It also includes my assessment for each project of whether a CIO with clinical training would have an advantage in managing it.

How have most organizations managed to cope without clinical chief information officers? They have invested in telecommunication networks; financial transaction systems; and order entry, results-reporting systems that physicians rarely use. They have not invested, yet, in clinical transaction and decision support systems that affect physicians in any substantive way. They have not actively invested in clinical decision support systems to give physicians advice in selecting and dosing pharmaceutical agents for patients or to give physicians counsel on their differential diagnoses for challenging patients. They have not introduced telemedicine networks. They have not created, or acquired, data warehouses of clinical and financial data for retrospective analysis of the quality and the outcomes of care. They have not introduced the use of risk-adjustment methodologies to control for the probabilities of patients' outcomes before treatment. Financial and marketing executives usually select case-mix systems without clinicians' active participation. They have not promoted the acquisition and use of computer-based patient records for physicians to use in their offices and in hospitals.

In other words, they have tended to avoid information and communication technologies that will directly affect physicians and have maintained traditional information systems departments concentrating on financially oriented accounting, inventory, scheduling, communication, and payroll systems. When physicians are directly affected by information or communication technology, lay vice presidents of information systems or chief information officers usually find clinicians to play the unofficial role of clinical information officer, to run interference for them and promote clinically oriented information technologies to clinicians. Shortly, almost all the investments made for information processing will be in clinically oriented information systems, and organizations will see the wisdom of hiring clinicians with formal training in health care informatics as chief information officers. In a health care organization, where the purpose of information systems increasingly will be to support and expedite the efficient and effective delivery of clinical care to patients, it is inconceivable that chief information officers will not be clinicians.

## Issues Facing CIOs of Most Integrating Health Care Organizations

| Issue | Importance of Clinical Experience |
|---|---|
| Selection of clinical transaction systems for basic clinical information collection and communication: laboratory, radiology, order entry and results reporting, enterprisewide scheduling, pharmacy. | Moderate |
| Selection of managed care information systems for PHOs, MSOs, and IPAs to allow them to manage inpatient and outpatient carve-out and capitation contracts and to collect data for retrospective study of physicians' practice habits. | Moderate |
| Selection of standardized office practice information systems to lead physicians to standard patient accounting and computer-based medical record systems. | High |
| Design and implementation of a wide-area communications network linking workstations in all facilities of the organization with standardized clinical and financial transaction systems. | Low |
| Design and implementation of a regional communications network linking physicians' homes and offices to electronic data about patients, electronic scheduling of services, and electronic mail to payers and other physicians. | High |
| Upgrading of financial information systems (primarily patient accounting) for management of managed care contracts. | Low |
| Procurement and implementation of computer-based patient records for intensive care units and emergency departments, the functional requirements of which may not be satisfied by patient care systems for hospitals. | High |
| Procurement and implementation of cost accounting systems for hospitals and group practices to enable managers to identify their "true" costs of operations. | Low |
| Design and implementation of a telemedicine network for communication by clinicians in real time and multimedia electronic mail to expedite clinical consultations. | High |
| Design and implementation of a home page, with derivative documents, on the Internet to be used by the community for access to general health information, details about clinicians, triage algorithms for patients, and schedules of clinical services. | Moderate |

## Issues Facing CIOs of Most Integrating Health Care Organizations *(continued)*

| Issue | Importance of Clinical Experience |
|---|---|
| Leadership for information systems planning and budgeting for the next five years. | High |
| Design, funding, and implementation of a relational corporate data warehouse to support retrospective data analysis for health services and clinical research. | High |
| Creation of a team of health services research specialists to analyze data from the data warehouse and support clinical data analysis and risk-adjustment by various managerial and clinical groups within the organization. | High |
| Tailoring of computer-based patient record systems to meet the needs of physicians, nurses, and others in ambulatory and inpatient settings. | High |
| Participation in managed care contracting initiatives to make certain that terms of contracts that affect information systems can be accomplished by the health care organization. | High |
| Development of training programs for all clinicians—physicians, nurses, physical therapists, pharmacists, and others—to learn to use computer-based patient records selected for office practices and inpatient settings. | High |
| Participation of the organization in national data collection initiatives, standardizing and producing data for national benchmarking programs (C/FIS of Voluntary Hospitals of America, IMSystem of JCAHO, HEDIS of NCQA, MQISS of HCFA, and PROs) devoted to accreditation, quality improvement, and outcomes management. | High |
| Definition of functional requirements and procurement of information systems, such as registries for cardiovascular surgery, cardiology, oncology, trauma surgery, and transplant surgery, for clinical departments of group practices and hospitals. | High |
| Standardization of software for electronic mail, groupware, and access to the Internet so that the organization can offer to its employees and on-line customers a standardized interface to all electronic information. | Low |
| Leadership of health services research staff for data analysis to support clinical quality improvement and outcomes management and practice guidelines development. | High |

# Chapter 5
## The Politics of Informatics

Why would a technophile such as I pick this title for a book chapter? At first light, it would appear that there is no relationship between politics and informatics. The former involves economics and income distribution and allocation of resources. The latter involves selection, implementation, and use of electronic information and communication systems to perform useful work in and across health care organizations. The former would appear to be the bailiwick of back-slappers and hand-shakers and baby-kissers. The latter would interest information systems departments and their technicians.

In fact, the successful selection, procurement, and implementation of information and communication systems is far more political than technical. Ignore the politics at your peril. Ignore the politics, and the technical issues will not matter, because implementation will fail and the potential benefits promised by the technology will not materialize. Attend to the politics, and deal with them, and which vendors your organization selects will not matter much, because, in a setting of consistent political interests, almost any vendor's product will perform well.

The politics of informatics may not appear to be crucial to what would seem to be technical procurements, such as those for transaction systems, communication networks, or data warehouses for retrospective analysis, but they determine the eventual success of those ventures in automation. Nowadays, providers are aggregating into larger organizations to take care of populations of people over time, and they want to share data about their patients electronically across political lines of group practices, hospitals, and other ambulatory treatment facilities and between departments within group practices and hospitals. Moving information about patients electronically takes far more standardization of data across those organizational boundaries than does the movement of paper records.

People are good at pattern recognition and can glean the information they need from paper records of all shapes and sizes, from text and images formatted in a wide variety of ways. Computers and communication networks fail at pattern recognition. They move information quickly, at minuscule marginal cost, provided the data are standardized and formatted exactly from one computer to another. Without that excruciatingly exact formatting, data cannot flow electronically from the laboratory system of a hospital to a communication network and into the computers in the offices of physicians. And those data will flow electronically only into the offices of physicians who have installed specific software, formatted just so, on their office computers to allow them to retrieve those data.

Frankly, it is amazing to me that technologies that move electrons and photons from place to place work at all, given the insight and flexibility inherent in people and absent in data processing equipment. So, because our health care communities want to move information about patients from one location of care to another electronically, standardization of those systems is necessary, and standardization introduces politics, across departments within institutions and between institutions.

What has brought politics into the process of selecting systems is that our interest in and need and capability for electronic communication of peoples' administrative and medical records within and between organizations have grown substantially. We have discovered networks. Electronic communication networks permit movement of data electronically from computer to computer, regardless of the distance between them, with incredibly low marginal costs, but with high start-up costs of standardization of data dictionaries, data formatting, network hardware and software, computer operating systems, and application programs. Because we tend to associate human capabilities with computers that do some things so much better than we can, such as sorting huge numbers of patients by name in seconds, we tend to underestimate the human effort required to set up computers to perform useful work, especially when more than one computer must share data with others across communication networks.

Politics tend to come into play when substantial resources must be allocated. Politics and economics are inextricably entangled. Within an institution with an influential director, politics may appear quiescent. The director considers rational arguments for this or that project and approves some and does not approve others. Life goes on, without interminable committee meetings in which people try to persuade others to their points of view about proper allocation of resources. A private practice of a single physician, or a small group practice with a single owner, may appear to be free of political wrangling over funds. Even a large group practice, hospital, or health plan with a dominant leader and a clear mission and goals may appear free of political tension. In those organizations, computer technologies may have been introduced in the past without dissension for financial accounting, and they probably work well. Even departmental clinical systems may work well. They perform their automated information management in specific departments—radiology, pharmacy, and laboratory—and produce paper reports that fill paper medical records.

A medical community including a solo physician's office, a small single-specialty group practice, a larger multispecialty group practice, and a hospital probably moves patient data between the provider organizations using paper records. Each of these organizations electronically calculates its bills for services it has performed in its own patient accounting system, and each produces claims forms that its patient accounting system prints on paper to mail to the health plans used by its patients. The hospital and larger group practice may send claims electronically to some payers, from their computers to the computers of those insurers over standard telephone lines. Provider organizations do not share financial risk for the care of those patients. They rely on fax transmissions of small documents and couriers for large medical records to move information about patients quickly from location to location.

Into this happy scene, introduce managed care and financial risk sharing among provider organizations. Now the pressure mounts among physicians and hospitals for cost control. Information systems remain departmental within the hospital and the group practices, and only paper is exchanged between them. Each organization reduces staff, and each saves money wherever it can by purchasing supplies and durable goods with more attention to their costs than they did before. And those initiatives work for a few years, while fees for services rise annually less than they did in the past. The physicians' practices and the hospital may contemplate sharing financial risk for capitated covered lives, but they retain financial independence, and each maintains its own patient accounting and financial management information systems. There may be tough negotiations between hospital and physicians over how to divvy up the pot of money they receive monthly from the health plan with whom they share financial risk, but they can handle those negotiations using paper reports from their financial systems to guide them.

At the same time, however, health plans demand more data from the physicians' practices about the screening procedures they perform on their patients, and health plans and state regulatory agencies demand more clinical data from hospitals about the treatment and outcomes of patients. Those data collection efforts require expensive manual chart review. Consequently, many physicians' practices and hospitals are considering automating their clinical record systems. While the physicians' practices and hospitals would not contemplate integrating their financial systems until they merge their organizations, they will consider sharing computer-based patient records.

Sharing electronic information between divisions of a single organization is difficult to accomplish, and nearly impossible between organizations. Ignore politics and doom the process to frustration and failure. Recognize politics, prepare for give and take about who pays for what in order to share data electronically across institutional boundaries, and the process of governance that necessarily must precede the process of technical selection and implementation can start.

Take the solo practice, the small single-specialty group, the larger multispecialty group, and the hospital to which we referred before. Imagine that someone in each organization simultaneously decides a computer-based patient record (CPR) would make patient care and quality improvement studies more efficient and effective. Each organization starts to define its requirements and to select a system.

The solo practice selects a system based on the MS-DOS operating system and creates its own database of clinical findings and treatments it will automate electronically. The small single-specialty group selects a system based on the UNIX operating system and creates its own database of clinical findings and treatments to automate, formatting data elements any clinician would collect in a different way from the solo physician and collecting many data elements not collected in the solo physician's system. The larger multispecialty group practice selects another vendor's system, using the VAX operating system, and derives a third formatting scheme for common data elements any clinicians would collect and many data elements unique to its practice. The hospital selects a fourth system, based on an IBM mainframe computer with an MVS operating system, and formats data in a fourth way.

Now each organization has a computer-based patient record, but they cannot share data electronically among them. Paper must continue to flow between their organizations to convey clinical and financial data, and each organization must pay part of the cost of duplicate data entry when data elements collected electronically in one organization, and then printed on paper, must be reentered electronically in a second organization to have those data in its CPR.

The best example involves laboratory results. For a physician to keep laboratory results in his or her office CPR that were originally obtained and stored electronically in the hospital, he or she must pay to have those data entered manually. For the hospital to include laboratory results obtained in the physician's office prior to admission in its CPR, they must be entered by hand in the hospital. Electronic interfaces between incompatible CPR systems are possible, but the wide variety of CPR systems available for office practices makes it highly impractical for a hospital to plan to write interfaces to all of those selected by physicians' practices without trying to standardize which systems they select. One of the principal reasons medical service organizations exist is to help standardize office practice CPR systems for physicians' offices, to permit them to share clinical data about patients electronically.

When organizations that want to share data electronically recognize that they cannot tell each other which information systems to select, or which data elements to put into those systems, but must plan the standards for those systems together to avoid hideous costs of retrofitting and interfacing incompatible systems, early recognition and introduction of a political process to resolve issues about who pays for standardization become paramount. If two group practices share one vendor's CPR system and want to share electronic data with a third practice, who pays for retrofitting data dictionaries and electronic interfaces between systems? Data elements must be standardized and electronic bridges must be written to convey data electronically between them. The trauma service of the hospital wants to acquire an electronic trauma registry to win accreditation as a regional trauma center. Who manages and funds standardization of the trauma registry so the data can flow electronically into it from the hospitals' main CPR system and from the trauma registry into the hospital CPR? You might say the hospital does, because the trauma center is part of the hospital, but the trauma center may have funding from external sources and may resist having to standardize its system with the hospital if a less expensive solution would satisfy the accrediting organization.

What process would you use to get multiple hospitals, multiple group practices, or both, which recently decided to manage populations of patients under a risk contract with a major insurer, to standardize their CPR systems so that records from one organization are available electronically at workstations of the other organizations? If a hospital's CPR system is perfectly adequate for that hospital but needs substantial modification to accept data electronically from a partner hospital or from group practices that have recently joined the integrating delivery system those organizations are forming, who pays for the modifications?

As a general rule, leaving funding for standardization up to the various operating units that express interest in sharing computer-based patient records dooms the planning project to failure or to accomplishments far short of expectations. Operating units, be they group practices or hospitals, will find countless excuses not to fund the standardization required to make shared CPR systems function successfully. They will frustrate adoption of standards in the first place by posturing to shift the burden of costs to other operating units. Each organization will argue for the adoption of standards for data elements, operating systems, application programs, and hardware that are closest to its own and that will require the least investment by it to accommodate.

So, are provider organizations that are not economically integrated doomed to failure when they consider planning for CPR systems in common? No, but they do have to address the politics of funding standardization first. They need to meet and agree on the general scope of their efforts. Are they agreed that they want to implement shared CPR systems that permit them to move data electronically from one location of care to another? Do they want to have most, if not all, clinical information about patients available electronically from all locations of care in their integrating delivery system? If they do, they need to create a planning organization of clinicians and managers from all the organizations to establish goals and standards for a shared system. It may take three to six months of periodic retreats, with staff work in between, to define their requirements.

The staff also needs to inventory existing computer systems, including communication networks, in all organizations to predict the costs of modifying or replacing them in order to collect and move standardized data from location to location. Senior executives of participating organizations need to understand the likely costs involved and agree to share the costs of standardization to minimize the otherwise interminable haggling over standards.

The standards for creation, display, and communication of documents on the World Wide Web (WWW) of the Internet, using hypertext markup language (HTML) and its successors, will enable health care organizations to share clinical information about patients much more easily than they have until now. The WWW has established a set of standards for movement of data over communication networks, and many corporations are using them to define the ways in which proprietary documents will move electronically between locations connected by their corporate networks. Functions to support data entry forms and multimedia database searching from workstations on the WWW appear and improve daily.

In the near future, international standards for community-based medical records, with acceptable security protections incorporated in the networks that convey the data, will be based on Internet standards. In the meantime, planning for CPR systems needs to involve multiple organizations and painful standardization of data elements and technology that require political will and foresight from the very beginning of planning. Most of the difficult decisions about implementing CPR systems are really capital allocation decisions that involve multiple operating units, and so they are inherently political. Recognize politics early in your planning efforts, so you do not meet with frustration and failure after much time wasted fantasizing about technical possibilities.

# Chapter 6

## All the News That's Fit for Bytes

I wake up lazily, refreshed, on a rainy Tuesday morning. It's the beginning of my vacation at the beach in Corolla, North Carolina. My children are watching television and playing board games. My wife is reading a book. I pour a cup of coffee and decide to check the news, but I don't want the news as the television and radio networks give it to me, homogenized and spoon fed, while I sit passively waiting for topics of interest, enduring subjects alternately appalling and boring and the noise of advertising. What a wasteful way to consume information, all of which is meant for the lowest common denominator—the American with an eighth grade education who devours soft drinks, detergent, and cake mix.

The information on television and radio is free, and I get what I pay for. I get information funded by advertising. The media are still mass-produced, with the same copy of information distributed daily, weekly, or monthly to every consumer. I want information specific to my interests in health care—informatics, managed care, and the economy. I want to know about the companies in which I have investments, not the thousand of others in which I do not. I'm not interested in more coverage of Bill Clinton and Monica Lewinsky; the fratricide in Bosnia; the latest atrocities to women's, gay, and minority rights; or who is sleeping with whom or addicted to what in Hollywood.

On this dreary morning, without the rush to the office to occupy myself, I want to determine the news content I receive, not what the medium (TV, radio, or newspaper) that presents it to me wants me to receive. I want to know the weather for my area south of Norfolk, Virginia, and north of Wilmington, North Carolina, and east of Raleigh, North Carolina. I want financial information on the industries and companies in which I have an interest. I want news for the sports teams I follow, not all the amateur and professional sports. I want headlines from major newspapers, with the opportunity to select any of them and read the full text of the stories.

CNN won't give it to me. Neither will CNBC. ESPN only shows me sports. The Weather Channel reports on weather, but usually for regions of the world where I am not located. The pharmacy 20 miles from here only carries *The Washington Post, The Raleigh News*, and the *Observer*. I want to be able to download information to my notebook computer from a news server on the Internet, giving me text and images on topics of interest that I can use as I would a newspaper, perusing it to my heart's content in my cottage, tethered by the electrical cable to my PC or, on the beach, relying on battery power. And I'd be willing to pay a monthly fee for such a service, at least as large as those I pay for general news media—the *Washington Post*, the *Wall Street Journal*, and cable television.

There is such an alternative, still relatively immature but preferable to the media designed for mass audiences—news customized to your interests and distributed over the Internet to your desktop or portable PC. It includes a browser software package to allow you to review the information at your leisure, in the order and depth you want to consume it. The service that downloads the data to your computer keeps it current throughout the day if you have a direct connection to the Internet, or updates the data whenever you log onto the Internet via a modem. Both the browser software and the service are free, funded by unobtrusive advertising. The *Wall Street Journal* and the *Washington Post* offer a personal edition electronically, giving the subscriber the opportunity to identify the types of stories desired, by subject matter.

The PointCast Network provides even more features: headlines and the political, business, and international news stories behind them; financial information from companies; weather details and maps from up to 50 cities around the globe; amateur and professional sports stories and statistics; and press releases and news by industry sector. I follow Computers/Electronic, Education, Health Care/Hospitals, Internet/Online, Medical/Pharmaceuticals, Publishing, Software, Stocks, Telecommunication and Television, and Lifestyle, with stories such as those found in the Style sections of newspapers and in *People, Time,* and *Money* magazines. I also read the contents of news stories (national and local) from the *Boston Globe, Los Angeles Times,* and *Washington Post.*

I can get the news I want, customized to the topics of interest to me, easily legible and searchable on my notebook computer in a rural and remote corner of North Carolina, at far less cost and inconvenience than driving into town for a newspaper. The word "searchable" is very important. You can't search the newspaper for text strings or references easily. You have to scan all the text, turning pages slowly and reading columns methodically. But when far more information is stored in computer text, you can search for words, strings of words, or strings of characters much more quickly.

Long before I can get the *Boston Globe,* I can read all the articles published this morning, including the local ones about school uniforms for public schools in Lawrence, Massachusetts. The text, created by a writer in Massachusetts, is sent electronically to the PointCast Internet server in California and is distributed via the Internet as a stream of bits to my computer, all in seconds and at negligible marginal cost.

In the pharmacy to which I could drive to buy a newspaper, I can only purchase the *Washington Post,* which does not include weather maps of the globe, or news from Boston or Los Angeles. And I'd still have to drive 20 miles back to my cabin in Corolla to enjoy reading the news in it with a fresh cup of coffee. Far better to make one short telephone call, connect to the Internet through my IAP (Internet access provider), and download data from the PointCast Network. In the future, the news will be delivered electronically, via telephone and cable television wires, directly into your personal computer. An early version of such a service is available for free from the PointCast Network. The *Wall Street Journal,* the *Washington Post,* and the *New York Times* also offer online, interactive electronic editions, but

*All the News That's Fit for Bytes* 37

you get content from one publisher and you may have to pay a monthly fee to have access to all the content.

So, how did I download the browser for the PointCast network and start using its service? I used Netscape Navigator, although I could have used Microsoft Internet Explorer just as easily, to visit the PointCast site on the Internet's World Wide Web (www.pointcast.com) and followed the instructions to download the software. Nothing could be easier. I could have visited the same site with the Internet connection through America Online, CompuServe, Prodigy, or the Microsoft Network.

Once my PC is on the Web, I can download the PointCast software to it. Once I have the executable file on my machine, I can run it and automatically install the PointCast software. It creates icons on my desktop in Windows 3.1, Windows 95, Windows 98, or Macintosh, whichever I use. When I click on the icon for the PointCast Network, the software searches for an Internet connection, either directly through a local area network or indirectly through a modem and dial-up connection. I have to establish a connection to the Internet before PointCast Network can download news to my computer. The software instructs me in ways to customize it to indicate topics of news and cities for weather information that I want. Downloading information takes seconds with a direct digital connection through a local area network in my office, and a few minutes by a dial-up connection through the modem in my notebook computer, using the telephone line in our cabin.

The PointCast Network, originally created as a joint venture between EDS (Electronic Data Sciences Corporation) and Time-Warner Communications, raised more than $30 million in an initial offering of common stock to the public. You might ask why the PointCast Network is attractive to the investor community if it is giving away its client software and news services. It is giving them away now to create a market for those services, just as Netscape and Microsoft give away their Internet browsers and as NBC gives away the nightly news on television. They want to build market share to attract advertising. PointCast Network is the first, but certainly not the last, application for the Web that distributes customized news for individual users. PointCast is not so much a producer of news as it is a distributor of news from many sources.

The network is financed by unobtrusive interactive advertising—if you see an ad for a product or service and want more information, you can click on the image and PointCast automatically connects you to the site on the Web where that product or service is more fully described. I saw an ad this morning, in the upper right-hand corner of the computer screen, while I was reading international news, about new Pontiac sports cars. I clicked on the image and PointCast launched Netscape Navigator, the browser for the Web that I prefer, and connected my computer to www.pontiac.com, where I could obtain more information. At the same time, PointCast Network noted that I chose to find out more about Pontiac cars, and Pontiac recognized another contact from PointCast Network.

Marketing via the Internet will be more precise and quantifiable than in print media. Publishers of printed materials can never say with certainty who gave attention to an advertisement, unless people send in a response card by mail or call a telephone number. With the Web, every time someone wants to learn more about General Motors cars or about products sold through the Sharper Image (two firms that advertise on PointCast Network), the advertiser's Web site receives a new contact. The company cannot identify the person as an individual user, but it can identify the Internet access provider—CompuServe, America Online, Netcom, or UUNET—through which the individual made the contact. Still, it's easier to gauge what types of advertising messages are most productive of consumer interest.

In summary, PointCast Network is available for you to use by downloading the PointCast Network software from the Web site. Try it and see if you like it. I am convinced it's a prototype of the way information will be distributed over the information superhighway in the future. Imagine getting the contents of medical publications of interest to you this way.

# Chapter 7
## Getting the Most Benefit from Information Systems Consultants

Consultants are usually well-meaning people who enjoy the variety of organizations and problems they face in their work. Most do not like to get bogged down in fruitless and wasteful consulting engagements any more than managers of health care organizations like to supervise them, but at least consultants are paid for their time. The health care organization that defines a project poorly, does not know what it wants from consultants, or does not direct consultants will pay the price in squandering of increasingly scarce resources. The tips in the following chapter for managing an information systems consulting engagement apply to most consulting engagements and to the use of other expensive advisers, such as attorneys and engineers. But information systems is a field particularly foreign, and often threatening, to most administrators and physician executives, so the risk of wasting money on unsuccessful consulting engagements is high.

Why use consultants? What role do they play in society, in general, and in information systems planning and procurement, specifically? In general, the U.S. business world is more complex than ever before, in terms of politics, economics, regulations, human resources, and technologies. Information systems fall into the latter category, in which new technologies, new vendors, and new functions appear every day. Most general managers need help in planning for, and implementing, information and communication systems often costing millions of dollars and affecting every employee and every customer of the organization. Consultants can reduce the time required to make a good decision and implement systems less expensively than the organization could accomplish on its own, because consultants know more about strengths and weakness of current technologies and vendors than most managers do. But they do not know your company as well as you do, and they probably don't know your business and your industry as well as you do. So you need to stay very involved to make certain that what they recommend, and help you implement, is what your organization really needs. Most of the problems organizations have with consultants derive from the managers themselves, who are not as involved in the process of defining requirements for information and communication systems and in implementation decisions as they need to be.

Consultants should transfer some of their skills to the organization that has retained them in the course of their engagement. They need to leverage their knowledge of technologies, vendors, and business requirements to help the organization obtain a good result faster and at less cost than it could on its own. They need to promote constructive change in the organization and to insist that the work rules and habits of employees change to get the best results from the new technology. Consultants worth their billings need to push the organization to take full advantage of the technologies it acquires. If that means reassigning employees, giving some new duties, or even relieving some of their duties, the organization should do so. Consultants with guts to disagree with those who retain them will be more valuable to you than those who passively follow your orders. If you have all the answers, you ought not have hired a consultant in the first place.

You will find that the simple tips below have much more to do with the governance of the organization seeking consulting advice than with the consultants themselves.

## Know What You Want to Do

Take the time to define your requirements for information systems and your requirements for a consultant as specifically as you can. Don't avoid starting for fear of making a mistake or neglecting something important. The exercise of first defining specifically what you want before you call in outsiders to tell you what they think you want is invaluable. Most health care leaders know what they want to do, but, when it comes to information systems, they may be less certain, because they probably do not understand the capabilities and limitations of the technologies available for licensing. This problem is compounded for health care managers who do not know anything about clinical care or medical records but who persist in trying to control the acquisition of clinical information systems they think will reduce the operating costs of their facilities. An example is the manager who decrees that a hospital will have a computer-based patient record (CPR), because with it he thinks he can automate clinical pathways and make the medical staff adhere to them. He may not understand the functions of CPRs that appeal to physicians, or that his facility lacks basic, standardized feeder systems required by any CPR to make it useful to clinicians.

## Have a Strategic Plan for the Organization That Defines the Functional Needs for Information Technologies

Many, maybe most, health care organization lack specific, detailed strategic and operating plans. The reason may be that most are tax-exempt and their leaders do not want to distress or alarm any of their many and varied constituencies by making detailed and explicit how they intend to spend their capital in the future. They do not want to admit which or how many insurers they will try to contact, with which and how many physicians they will partner to form PHOs or HMOs, or which medical groups they will try to acquire. They want to be all things to all people. That is the way with tax-exempt, "charitable" institutions, but it leads to squandering much time and effort on committee meetings to build consensus about each management issue facing them. Consequently, it is difficult for them to plan successfully for their information systems needs. Information needs must be tied directly to explicit needs and wants of the organization, defined in a strategic plan. Without an organizational strategic plan, one cannot produce a specific organizational strategic information systems plan that will direct the information systems staff to allocate capital effectively. Yet, most information systems directors are told to plan for information systems, not knowing what the organization truly wants. Imagine planning for a hospital information system without knowing if hospital leaders will emphasize or de-emphasize managed care, PHO development, acquisition of group practices, sharing clinical and financial data among member institutions, marketing centers of excellence, or promoting specific clinical "product lines," or even knowing whether they intend to sell their hospitals and move into the HMO business.

**Have an Organizational Structure That Indicates Who Is in Charge, and How Much Capital He or She Can Spend on Any Information Systems Projects**
Information systems projects cost a lot of money, often tens of millions of dollars for a major new information system in a large hospital or a group practice with hundreds of physicians. Too often, planning projects for information systems start de novo, without clear responsibility for planning or for authority to spend the money to procure a system once requirements have been defined and a process has been chosen for satisfying them. Many organizations have multiple planning groups working simultaneously on projects that will affect one anothers' plans, but without any coordination or clear authority. For instance, I know of one system that allowed three hospitals each to plan for digital storage systems for medical records, but no planning occurred to make certain the hospitals (in one system) adopted the same vendor's product or that the images from the system would be legible on workstations attached to the organization's wide-area network. I know of another organization that had three committees working simultaneously, one on an information systems plan (without a corporate strategic plan, by the way), one on procurement of a computer-based patient record for some (but not all) of the system's facilities (this committee was led by administrators, not physicians), and one on physicians' workstations. The committees were doomed to failure because they were not coordinated and had no corporate commitment, in the form of a strategic plan, a strategic information systems plan, or a budget, to support their efforts or give their recommendations authority.

**Do Not Be Afraid to Interview Fellow Managers and Physician Leaders Yourself**
Much of the early work of consultants is spent in interviewing people in the organization to find out what they want and expect from information systems. These interviews cost a lot of money, because the consulting firms usually charge more than $1,000 per day for relatively young and inexperienced junior employees to perform the interviews, and they separate the managers who hired the consultants from their own constituents. I believe the interviews need to be done by information systems staff themselves, with notes from those interviews transcribed into a document that fairly summarizes the answers and opinions of those interviewed. The interviews need to be conducted with a broad segment of the people likely to be affected by a proposed information system. If the interviews are meant to help the organization define its strategic information systems plan, the people interviewed should have read the latest detailed, explicit organizational strategic plan. If the organization does not have such a plan, do not waste time and money organizing interviews to find out what senior managers and physicians want from information systems. Use the interviews to start the process of creating the organizational strategic plan.

**If You Must Hire Consultants to Write the Strategic Information Systems Plan for Your Organization, Hire Them Carefully**
Consultants can twist whatever they hear in their interviews inside the organization into a list of preferences (functional requirements) that lead to exactly the sort of information systems they understand. Worse, some consultants will lead their clients to select information systems they know how to implement and install. Hiring a certain consulting firm may

accurately predict that, several years later, the organization will install systems the consulting firm already knows best. Worse, some firms with large staffs trained for systems development are much more likely to recommend software development, because no vendor will meet the precise needs of the client organization. Software development usually is much more expensive in time and money than the client organization expects when it signs up to create a system. Agree to software development as a last resort, after you are certain that no vendors will meet your needs and that your needs are so pressing and strategically important that meeting them justifies the expense and risk of development. Generally, it is much more prudent for an organization to license existing software from a reputable vendor and to contract with that vendor to enhance its systems in specific ways than to take on the very uncertain task of creating an entirely new system. Talk to many references on any consultants you are considering hiring, especially if you will entrust your strategic information systems plan to them and you suspect they may lead you toward custom development.

### Define Functional Requirements in as Specific a Way as Possible

Consultants may be very helpful in this effort, because they should have on file detailed reports of functional requirements by type of business requiring automation. If they don't have such reports or want to create a new set of reports for your organization, consider switching to consultants who have faced, and managed well, a similar project for another health care organization. You want to pay for as little on-the-job training of neophyte consultants as you can. Let other organizations with money to burn do that.

### Know How Consultants Differ from One Another and Hire a Firm that Fits Your Requirements

Consultants vary in their skills, of course. Learn about the strengths of the various firms you consider. Firms that specialize in "strategy" would worry me if they do not also have strong expertise in application programs, telecommunications, and implementation. Strategy is a safe haven for the young firm without extensive resources. You might find them naive about the details of your business or about the vendors you eventually consider. After all, God *and* the devil are in the details.

Some consultants specialize in one type of information system, such as patient accounting applications for hospitals, general ledger systems, telecommunication networks, laboratory systems, or group practice accounting systems. Hire a firm that understands your needs well, and don't hire a firm your organization knows and likes if the project you want it to consult on is outside of its expertise. Some are skilled in contract negotiation with vendors and promise to more than cover their fees by the savings they can negotiate for you with vendors. Be wary of them if you want a consultant to find a suitable vendor for your organization, because they might lead you to vendors who they know charge exorbitant prices initially and discount generously in negotiations.

Selecting a system requires knowing the industry you are in and your needs, not which vendor will give the largest discounts. Separate the selection of a vendor and product from negotiation of contract terms with that vendor. Some consultants really are not interested in procurement of vendors' systems, because they want to build systems from scratch. Selecting such a consultant for your procurement may lead you down the primrose path to software development. Be wary, and ask consultants about all their projects, what they do, what they prefer to do, and what they have done, for whom. Then call their clients.

Some consultants are far more technical and do good work in installing software, while others do better work helping the organization create a detailed information systems plan. Again, ask in detail about what they do and where their expertise lies. If they say they can do it all and you retain them, study them closely to make certain your organization is not paying $1,000-$1,500 per day for junior members of the firm to learn to do "it all" at your site.

**Make Certain You Know before You Contract with a Consultant Who Will Be the Day-to-Day Manager of Your Consulting Engagement**

Too often, firms fly in their very best presenters, with the most knowledge of your industry and, perhaps, of your firm and your competitors, and they list those luminaries as members of the consulting team to work on your project. Once their firm wins the contract, you see those luminaries little, if ever, again, because they are off presenting at other potential clients, and your project is managed by someone much younger and less experienced in your business and your requirements than you are. You need to be comfortable that the day-to-day manager of your engagement knows what he or she is doing, because that person will be your contact with the luminaries of the firm and will be the eyes and ears of the entire firm at your site. Consequently, if the consultant does not see or hear something important to your organization's eventual success with an information systems project because of lack of experience or expertise, your project, your organization, and you suffer.

**Be as Specific as Possible in Defining the Work Plan for a Consultant, and Do Not Let the Consultant Write It**

Consultants know far better than you do how they make money on engagements, what their strengths and weaknesses are, and who will or won't be assigned to your project. They want you to be specific in your requirements for information systems. They do not necessarily want you to be specific in your requirements of them. If you do not specify in detail what you expect from them, how will you know when the engagement is done? How will you know when you have received your money's worth from them? Make certain you define your expectations in detail, including the depth of detail expected in any document they produce for you. If consultants are building a system for you, make certain it is well documented, so you can continue to work on the system with employees after the consultants have left your organization. Too often, consultants cobble together software that is poorly documented and you need to use them to continue the project.

**It Pays to Know What You Want and Expect from Consultants**

Good consultants will want the same thing you do. They don't want to waste their time in frustrating engagements that accomplish nothing because the organization did not have its priorities sorted out ahead of the engagement. Good consultants are so busy that they want clearly defined engagements so they can succeed, earn their money, and leave a satisfied client behind to produce good references.

# Chapter 8
## The Future of Computers

In November 1971, Intel, a small start-up company, announced the first microprocessor—the Intel 4004. It used solid-state integrated circuit technology that the firm had been using to make memory "chips" to develop the logic circuitry of a computer's central processing unit. A tiny company in the land of the gold rush, where most dreams of fortune never materialized, Intel was not likely to threaten the titans of computer manufacturing, such as IBM, which was growing at a torrid pace to meet the demand for its System 360 business computing systems.

Less than 25 years later, computing products made with the microprocessor progeny of the Intel 4004 would overwhelm IBM in the marketplace and lead it to lose more than $8 billion in a single year and start a process to cut more than 100,000 employees from its work force. By then, most of IBM's product lines and computing platforms, from equipment for secretaries to its fastest supercomputers, had already embraced microprocessor technology, but the organization still thought of itself synonymously with big blue mainframes that the microprocessor had miniaturized.

Today, supercomputers are parallel processing machines, in that they are made of parallel arrays of microprocessors. In 1994, an Intel Paragon supercomputer made of about 1,024 Pentium microprocessors became the world's fastest computer, achieving more than 280 billion floating point operations (gigaflops) per second. In September 1995, Intel and Sandia National Laboratories announced a contract with the Department of Energy to create a Paragon supercomputer with more than 8,000 Pentium Pro microprocessors that would surpass 1.8 trillion floating point operations (1.8 teraflops) per second.

In the December 1996 issue of *Byte* magazine, the microprocessor was described as "the life-support system for the modern world." Not a bad performance for a device born only 25 years ago. Today, there is far more gold in Silicon Valley, south of San Francisco, than was ever found in the mountains east of Sacramento.

## The Pace of Change
In the next five to 10 years, the pace of technological improvement in microprocessors will accelerate, and so will concomitant enhancements to the performance of computers that contain them. Intel and its competitors, including IBM, will continue to make more efficient microprocessors, and computer manufacturers will include parallel arrays of microprocessors in their equipment. Of the likelihood that technological improvements in microprocessors will decline or stop, Mark Bohr, a research fellow at Intel, told *Byte* magazine in April 1996, "There's no sign of the technology slowing down. If we're going to run into a wall, it's more than 10 years out." The technological "wall" he refers to is a physical inability to condense more microscopic transistors onto microprocessor space.

In the same issue of *Byte* magazine, John Kelly, a Vice President with IBM, said that "with CMOS (complementary metal-oxide semiconductor) technology and a lot of hard work, in a decade we'll be using x-ray lithography and other techniques to deliver a (micro)processor that has 50,000,000 to 100,000,000 transistors and operates at 1 gigahertz (1 billion cycles per second)." For comparison, the current Pentium Pro microprocessor includes 5.5 million transistors and operates at 200 megahertz (200 million cycles per second), and the Pentium II microprocessor includes about 8 million transistors and operates at 400 megahertz. That's a lot of room for improvement!

Not only are microprocessors improving in calculating speed, they are also improving in multimedia capabilities. The MMX Pentium and Pentium II chips from Intel will be sold in versions with clock cycle speeds up to 400 MHz, optimized for multimedia computation, to handle high-resolution images, video, and high-fidelity sound more efficiently and effectively. The MMX instruction set improves video and audio performance two- to fourfold and can render three-dimensional graphics that compare favorably with specialized graphics microprocessors. For routine processing of data files and numerical calculations, the MMX is about 10 percent faster than earlier Pentium chips with the same clock speeds. Improvements in processing video and audio signals will enhance the performance of computers with the MMX microprocessors in rendering multimedia content for education, entertainment, and video conferencing. All Pentium II microprocessors incorporate the MMX instruction set.

The Internet's World Wide Web is more demanding of multimedia processing than the text-based Internet and business networks used by most people today. But the World Wide Web is the future. The MMX microprocessor was designed for computer games that involve high-resolution graphics and sound and for multimedia education and conferencing. The personal computer is becoming the window to the multimedia digital world of cyberspace. Microprocessors will continue to improve from one generation to the next to make cyberspace as realistic as possible, and with their improving capabilities will come myriad applications for health care services, either not cost-effective or not even contemplated until now.

## Microelectronics Improving Faster Than Expectations
We need to drop our preconceived notions about how much computing power and communication capability cost. Those expenses will continue to decline as new features and functions are added to personal computers and as computers become lighter, more portable, more communicative, and more capacious for storing digital data. For instance, in 1974, the Intel 8080 microprocessor delivered one million instructions per second (1 MIPS) for $1,250. A little

# The Future of Computers

more than 20 years later, Intel's Pentium Pro microprocessor delivered 1 MIPS for about $1. The cost of computing, estimated in the price of a million instructions per second, fell by more than three orders of magnitude in those 22 years.

The price of storing one thousand bytes of data in computer random access memory has fallen in the past 12 years from $15 per kilobyte to less than one cent per kilobyte. The price of permanent magnetic data storage has fallen from $220 per megabyte to three cents per megabyte in the past 12 years. The price to store a megabyte of data on an optical disk will reach one cent with digital versatile disks that are the same size and appearance of CD-ROM disks but that store more than 20 times as much data, about 16 gigabytes (16 billion bytes). The cost for a three-minute long-distance telephone call from New York to London has declined from $250 in 1930 to less than 10 cents today. With the deregulation of the telecommunication and cable TV industries and with widespread replacement of copper cable with fiberoptic cable that carries far more data at far lower cost, the price of communication will fall even more dramatically in the next few years.

## Improvements in Information Systems Lag

We would expect vendors of information systems to take advantage of the increasing efficiency of microcomputer data processing and to improve their software as fast as they can. Instead, vendors are selling old, inflexible systems because they do not have the capital to adapt them to newer technologies and because they have substantial numbers of clients whom they are maintaining on their existing systems at considerable profit. Vendors take far longer than we would wish to incorporate modern technologies into their products. For instance, most of the vendors of patient accounting systems have not incorporated any of the following technologies: powerful microprocessors and parallel processing systems, relational database management systems, and networks that adhere to the standards of open systems.

If they use personal computers for client machines, they are only window dressing for emulating dumb terminals. Most of the processing is still performed on the server. They do not incorporate relational database management systems that make modifying systems and extracting data more efficient—they maintain their rigid hierarchical databases designed for the first version of their software. They maintain proprietary networks rather than adopting open systems.

Vendors design their systems for one collection of hardware and software, and then they do not have the capital or incentive to rewrite their systems for better architectures that come shortly afterward. Microsoft, with billions of dollars in the bank for research and development, is trying to rewrite its client software now that network computing on the World Wide Web has become so important. Microsoft has the wherewithal to make the transition. Few other organizations developing information systems, and none serving the health care industry, have the capital to modify their existing systems so quickly. The incremental improvements they make to their products simply do not keep up with the rapid changes in the hardware and networking standards with which they must try to keep pace.

## What Health Care Leaders Need to Do about These Trends

As a leader of an organization, one who approves substantial budgets for information technology, you must ask yourself what new products and services these startling technological advances will create. How will they change health and medical care? Physician executives need to consider these subjects because they must guide spending on information technologies and how those technologies are used for the benefit of patients and the competitive advantage of their organizations.

In 1960, the cost to lease an IBM 7090 mainframe, with vacuum tubes instead of transistors in its memory and logic circuits, was about $20,000 per month. The cost of the personnel to manage that 7090 was about $2,000 per month. The hardware was 10 times more expensive than the personnel. Back then, we learned that computers were expensive and people were cheap. Now the reverse is the case. Computing technology is cheap, and getting cheaper, while payroll costs rise every year with inflation. Unfortunately, more than 35 years later, we still tend to invest too little in information technology and squander money in payroll costs for tasks that could be automated.

A powerful personal computer costs about $3,500 now and is capable of processing speeds and storage capacity (RAM and hard disk memory) greater than the mainframes of 10 years ago, let alone the 7090 of 1960. You can lease such a PC for about $200 per month. The person using that computer costs the organization at least $2,000 per month and as much as $10,000 per month. Senior executives who might use such a computer to expedite their work, if they knew how, cost their organizations much more per month. So the personal computer now costs the organization one-tenth to one-fiftieth the expense of the person who uses it.

You must lead your organization—where payroll costs are such a large and growing proportion of total operating costs—in identifying ways to improve the productivity of employees and affiliated physicians with practical, prudent, and imaginative deployment of computers, software, and networks. A helpful way of thinking about such issues is to imagine what processes in your organization you'd like to automate if automation were free. Of course, nothing is free, but the costs of digital data processing are falling faster than expectations for digital data processing are rising.

Our thinking habits, more than the technologies themselves, limit our ability to conceive of many functions that could be automated to the benefit of patients, organizations, families, and ourselves. We assume we cannot do what we have not seen done before. We need to look for solutions. If microprocessors are involved, the likelihood of finding a solution is improving annually at a stunning rate. What we can imagine today, we can afford next year and will take for granted the year after that. Let your imagination run freer than you usually permit it, and see what clinical or administrative functions you wish to automate. Then look for products and services to perform those functions.

## Some Examples

For instance, not long ago we used the DOS prompt to launch an application (word processing, spreadsheet, database, patient accounting system). We could have only one application operating at a time. We typed our print commands in arcane terms at the C:> prompt. A mouse was only a rodent.

Now we enjoy graphical interfaces and point and click with mechanical mice on intuitive icons and menus. We can keep simultaneously operating our scheduling, patient accounting, word processing, and electronic mail systems, and flip between them at the blink of an eye. In addition to text, we can store images, video, graphics, and sounds in our applications, such as our presentations. We can receive faxes at the same time we print our presentations and search the Internet's World Wide Web. We can use speech recognition to enter our commands, dictate our radiology interpretations, and complete our letters.

None of those functions we take for granted now was available 10 years ago. The World Wide Web was known to only a few people a few years ago. Now, we are beginning to understand that it will give us the standards we have heretofore lacked for multimedia document exchange and interactive data sharing between computers in health care. All these improvements have occurred because of the maturation of microprocessors and related technologies. Today, we can hear about a new computer-based patient record one minute and the next be operating a demonstration version of it over the Web. We can search the entire Medline database for key words and phrases in one or more of 30 medical lexicons in seconds from our homes, our offices, in fact, from anywhere on earth that has a telephone network to which we can connect by modem.

## What's Next?

Can you imagine major improvements in a number of areas of medical management and clinical practice from inexpensive computing and communication technologies? What would you think about the following options?

- Computer-based patient records with structured data entry using voice recognition.
- Expert systems for predicting treatment outcomes of patients.
- Telemedicine sessions between clinicians from their workstations.
- Home treatment counseling of patients and health plan members with interactive, multimedia, Web-based programs maintained on your practices' Web servers.
- Continuous monitoring of patients' vital signs, blood oxygen saturation, electrolytes, serum glucose, and myriad other physiological parameters over dedicated telephone lines via the Web.
- Automated interpretations of ECGs, EEGs, pap smears, and radiology studies by personal computers.

How about three-dimensional representations of detailed human anatomy that students can analyze on their clinical workstations; three-dimensional simulations of colonoscopy and cardiac catheterization; three-dimensional renderings of the molecular structure of enzymes and their receptors; or calculating the explanatory statistics that will predict the treatment outcome for a patient on the basis of preexisting patient characteristics? All these functions, which depend on fast microprocessors for acceptable performance, exist today either in commercial products or in informatics laboratories.

It may help to know that, as computer performance improves, most of the enhancements are absorbed by the human-computer interface. In 10 years, we have moved from text-based interfaces, with which users had to type arcane commands at line prompts, to graphical interfaces such as Apple Macintosh, Microsoft Windows, and IBM OS/2. There are other graphical interfaces, including NeXT Step from NeXT (acquired by Apple for $400 million) and Solaris from SUN Microsystems (which also created the Java programming language for the Internet).

The next step forward in user functionality will be reliable and affordable speaker-independent voice recognition. That technology is maturing rapidly and operating well on desktop PCs under IBM OS/2 Warp 4.0. Technology to rival it will be incorporated into Microsoft Windows and Macintosh OS in the late 1990s. Vendors of computer-based patient records for ambulatory care with whom we have spoken admit they are changing their client computer operating systems from Windows to OS/2 to take advantage of IBM's lead in voice recognition that is native to the OS/2 Warp 4.0 operating system. Microsoft hopes to stop much of that migration from Windows to OS/2 with the speech recognition feature in Windows 98.

## What about Video Conferencing?

We participate in multiple telephone conversations every day, usually making more than 10 calls daily at work, fewer from home. There are more than 250,000,000 long distance telephone calls each day in the United States and many more local calls. I would prefer to see, as well as hear, those persons with whom I have a relationship or want to establish one. For calls to people with whom I will have no relationship, to directory assistance or to a theater for its schedule, I do not need to see the person with whom I speak. Presuming that a video call is more expensive than a voice call, I'd rather use voice only for those brief calls to people who remain anonymous to me. But I'd prefer video calls with people I know, or want to know.

We have inexpensive cameras and multimedia personal computers that can present video now. Most new notebook computers with MMX Pentium and Pentium II microprocessors have the circuitry needed for MPEG (Motion Picture Experts Group) 2 coding and decoding of video and audio signals. In the next few years, most Americans in urban areas will be offered ADSL (asymmetric digital subscriber line) modems from telephone companies for about $50 per month. A workstation with such a modem can receive data over standard telephone wires at three to five million bits per second and send data at 500,000 bits per second (hence the name asymmetric), which is plenty of bandwidth for two-way video and audio teleconferencing.

To compete, the cable TV companies will offer modems providing up to 30 million bits per second downstream into our computers and about 400,000 bits per second upstream from our computers, also adequate bandwidth for bi-directional video and audio teleconferencing. The cable companies will lease those modems for $50 per month or less.

## How Will Microprocessors Affect Health Care?

Microprocessors of every sort are affecting medical care. Not only are they the essential components of personal computers and workstations that are increasingly appealing to use, but they are also embedded in the controls of infusion pumps, digital thermometers, remote pharmaceutical dispensers on patient care units, imaging equipment of all sorts, home monitoring equipment, anesthesia machines, ventilators, laboratory clinical chemistry machines, and automatic pap smear analyzers. Think of the tasks that are automated now, with primitive interfaces, and how cheaper personal computers with graphical interfaces and speech recognition could help to make them more useful. Think of all those information management tasks that could be automated with the right equipment and networks to benefit patients, health plan members, staff, and physicians. The faster microprocessors bring with them calculation speeds to support voice recognition, expert systems, high-resolution three-dimensional rendering of data, rapid conversion of analog audio and video signals to digital format, and other capabilities.

*The Future of Computers* 51

You will register and schedule patients with voice responses. You will contract with health plans for capitation payments, guided by expert systems. You will accept responsibility for health promotion and prospective medicine for health plan members assigned to your organization and will influence their demand for health care services with an extended Intranet, running on a Web server they can access over regular telephone lines using unique identification numbers and passwords. You will take and record histories and physicals on hand-held, backlit personal computers with touch screens for entering data. You will order diagnostic studies, perform procedures, and evaluate the results of diagnostic studies on hospitalized patients from your portable computer in your home or in your hotel when you travel.

You will teach patients how to prepare for procedures, what to expect from ailments, how to minimize their disabilities and recuperate most quickly, and how to prevent recurrences of injury or illness, with multimedia instructional programs on your Web server that they can access any time. You will prescribe medications and send prescriptions electronically from your office practice system. You will collect functional status data on patient outcomes, study clinical data on your processes of care, and compare your performance to that of other clinicians in your specialty using data from NCQA, JCAHO, state and federal government agencies, and cooperative payers that are stored in a relational database management system.

You will peruse clinical publications and complete continuing education from the monitor on your multimedia portable computer. You will manage human and inanimate resources of your medical practice with a sophisticated office practice management system to maximize operational efficiency. You will communicate and negotiate with payers and patients to obtain all the funds rightfully owed to the practice via electronic text and voice mail from your workstation on your office network. You will calculate and complete records due to regulatory agencies for certification and licensure and to federal and state agencies for tax purposes and will send them electronically according to EDI (electronic data interchange) standards.

Some aspect of each of these tasks will benefit from automation on a personal computer with a fast microprocessor. Many of them, especially the simulations and database analyses, will use the additional capabilities of readily available parallel processing systems to full advantage. The common World Wide Web browsers allow standardized information exchange of multimedia documents. With the advent of the Java programming language, information exchange is becoming more interactive and engaging, and the Web may well evolve into the standard architecture for modern computer-to-computer data exchange. In the process, the multimedia personal computer will become as much a communications device as a calculator or typewriter, and we will begin to use the Web for research, education, and teleconferencing.

In the near future, ever-improving microprocessors, either alone or in parallel arrays inside personal computers, will make the multimedia interfaces of personal computers much more intuitive, engaging, and easier to use. The personal computer is becoming a communications device just as a global multimedia network, the Internet, is evolving to receive it. The results will be functionality in administrative and clinical systems not considered possible before and far more potent ways of examining, treating, and teaching patients and health plan members than those used today. Leaders of health care organizations need to direct their organizations to anticipate improvements in workstations and networks and to pressure vendors to incorporate those technologies into their products as quickly as possible.

# Chapter 9
# The Future of Health Care Information Systems

What does the future hold for health care information systems? The forecast in general terms is certain. The inexorable movement to digital documents from paper ones will continue unabated. In fact, the advent of the World Wide Web of the Internet expedites the fundamental conversion from analog to digital documents. We will see fewer pens and more keyboards, mice, and light pens. We will use monitors more often to read results in digital format, and we will retrieve information less often from paper records. Physicians will enter orders directly into computers more often, and they will write orders on paper forms to be entered in electronic order entry systems by data terminal operators less often. Clinicians will urge patients to check their Web sites for detailed instructions on finding a location for care, preparing for a procedure, or managing an ailment. Members of the public will turn to the Web to learn to manage their symptoms, learn more about a disease, find preventive measures appropriate for age and sex, retrieve laboratory test results, or check on the reputation of a physician or a hospital.

Clinicians also will collect standardized information about their patients, and health plan members assigned to their care, so they can study the outcomes of their processes of care retrospectively. The Era of Accountability predicted in 1988 by Relman[1] has arrived. Ellwood's[2] call for large databases for the systematic study of the efficacy and the effectiveness of community medical practices has been answered by health care organizations, payers, regulatory agencies, and local governments that are building clinical and financial data warehouses. American Medical News contains lead articles about widespread interest in data warehouses and data mining among health care organizations, and the emergence of "managerial epidemiology" to identify best clinical outcomes and best practices from huge databases of observational data.[3,4]

Most of us involved in medical care believe the Socratic dictum[5] that tells us the unexamined life is not worth living. Most of the world's great philosophers would concur that the highest attainment of man is self-knowledge, or truth about oneself.[6] Now, consider the unexamined clinical practice. Is it worth performing? Does it benefit patients? Is it cost-effective? Is it safe? Does it warrant reimbursement by the federal government, or by other payers? How can we answer these questions if the practice is unexamined? If it is unexamined when paid for by fee-for-service, will it be unexamined when paid for by capitation? Does the way we finance care affect our concern for the cost-effectiveness of care? Would we scrutinize the efficacy and the efficiency of a treatment when paid by fee-for-service with the same zeal we would do so if our work were paid by capitation?

To answer these questions, we must examine our practices of caring for patients. Consider the wide variation in care among homogeneous neighboring communities that Wennberg[7-9] discovered in his studies. Does that variation warrant systematic study to find an explanation? Most of us would agree that clinical practices, even those in vogue, need scientific validation—certainly before they are practiced on us. Most of us would agree that wide variation in care deserves study to determine the multiple factors associated with the variation and to reduce variation that is not attributable to differences in patients.

How do we make this Socratic dictum more relevant to medical care? Money talks. Put providers at financial risk for the care of a population of people over time, and they will search for ways of reducing their costs of clinical care. Other industries have learned, from Deming,[10] Juran,[11] and Crosby,[12] among others, that reducing variation in a production process will help to increase the reliability of that process and reduce the operating costs associated with it. Reduction in process variability in health care services, according to Berwick,[13] means creating guidelines and interesting physicians and other clinicians in following them. Patients vary, so treatments should vary. Most of us would agree, however, that two similar patients should not receive two very different treatments if one treatment has demonstrably better results in most patients than the other. We would hope the health care professions would identify the most effective and efficient of the two alternatives and publicize to their peers which of the two treatments works best for the majority of patients.

Unfortunately, medicine is complicated, each patient is different; physicians learn different processes of care in different decades of study and in different places of training and have different prior clinical experiences that influence their choices of treatment for patients considerably. Eddy documented the presence of, and reasons for, wide variation in clinical care in his essays in the Journal of the American Medical Association published in the mid-1990s, and later collected into a book titled *Clinical Decision Making: From Theory to Practice.* "The plain fact is that many decisions made by physicians appear to be arbitrary—highly variable, with no obvious explanation. The very disturbing implication is that this arbitrariness represents, for at least some patients, suboptimal or even harmful care."[14]

Is the solution to the variability in medical practice really as simple as systematic study of observational data, profiling of physicians' practice habits with those data, education of those physicians in ways in which they differ from established practice guidelines and the practices of their peers, adoption of practice guidelines that produce the best outcomes, and continued collection and analysis of observational data? Yes and no. To paraphrase the Song of Solomon, there is nothing new under the sun. Education and progress have always been about comparisons, comparisons of the results of one established process with those of another. The one that produces the better outcomes tends to win favor over time, until a better process replaces it.

In health care, the providers of care, those who determine the processes of clinical care, the physicians, are many, largely unorganized, and unfamiliar with the practice habits, and their consequences, of other physicians of the same specialty. Physicians may study published literature, but usually they have not even a vague idea of what proportion of physicians like them practice in a similar way. Physicians have choices to prescribe medications, diets, and/or surgery for most ailments. Economic influences on physicians play a substantial role in affecting their clinical practices.

Promising technologies, the use of which benefit the physician economically, tend to receive earlier adoption than equally promising technologies that do not benefit financially the physician who prescribes them. New procedures and diagnostic tests, lucrative for the physicians who master their use, receive eager early adoption by those physicians of entrepreneurial spirit. Witness the extraordinary, and many would say excessive and hazardous, proliferation of liposuction centers and liposuctionists with dubious training.[15] Radial keratotomy has enjoyed a similar boom. Physicians struggling with forced discounting of their "bread and butter" procedures by managed care contracts have turned to elective cosmetic procedures for which they receive more pay for their time, directly from the patients themselves. Many studies, by Brook,[16,17] his colleagues,[18-20] and others have questioned the frequency with which lucrative elective procedures, such as cardiac catheterization and revascularization, carotid endarterectomy, total hip replacement, lower and upper gastrointestinal endoscopy, are performed.

Now our medical-industrial complex—providers of care and producers of therapeutic and diagnostic materials and equipment—can produce more goods and services than any western country can afford. Medical care is a preferred good, so, as people become more affluent, they tend to spend a larger proportion of their discretionary income on medical care.[21] Insurers and employers introduced managed care to contain the insatiable appetite of patients and providers for ever greater sums of money for medical care services. Managed care wins for payer discounts off the usual and customary fees of providers, but it does little to change processes of care. Many of the administrative interventions introduced to control clinical practice in the 1980s (second surgical opinion, utilization review, prior approval for procedures, claims adjudication for fraud and abuse) have squeezed some variation in care out of the health care system. Now payers turn to financial risk-sharing with providers to continue to reduce the rate of growth in health care costs. Provider organizations that take financial risk for the care of populations of people over time must concentrate on managing those costs as the way to make a profit. Ironically, most capitated providers do not want to collect or submit encounter data to payers, but, without them, they cannot measure their own performance to find opportunities to reduce variation in care among themselves.

Some regional payers have the capital and the opportunity to create for the providers with whom they contract for health care services the kinds of information systems those providers will need to manage risk successfully. Those payers can create extranets (Internet-based networks using public telephone connections between computers and various security methods to protect the privacy of communications), shared data warehouses, and standardized transaction systems for their affiliated physicians. They can become indispensable to their contracting providers by giving them the architecture and the features of information systems those providers will need to manage risk successfully. Payers can obtain laboratory results for beneficiaries from reference laboratories where the studies are performed; radiology interpretations from radiology groups contracted to perform diagnostic radiology services; prescription data from pharmacy benefit plans; and claims and encounter data from contracting providers. They can create relational data repositories that can serve as electronic medical records for their beneficiaries. The electronic records can include problem lists, fashioned from diagnosis codes on claims data.

For a regional payer to create an electronic record for a medical community, it must lead those providers in the selection of standards for electronic information exchange that medical communities usually lack when they try to create electronic medical records to be shared among themselves. Providers have a very difficult time establishing standards for information sharing, because they usually cannot agree on how to distribute the cost of standardization among themselves. The payer can fill the leadership void with a single voice, set the standards, establish the architecture, and offer the network to providers at low cost. Physicians and hospitals will begin to use the medical record, find it expedites their work and saves them money, and become dependent on it. The payer can charge modest transaction fees that eventually add to a handsome return on its investment in the network. Providers may be only vaguely aware that the payer has made itself indispensable to them by its contribution to information management systems on which they depend.

Perhaps this vignette signals an emerging role for regional payers. As providers organize to take financial risk, payers can mature from the role of third-party administrators and insurers processing claims to providers of communication and information systems to anneal providers together into delivery systems. In the world of unfettered fee for service, payers insured employers against the costs of health care services for their employees and dependents. When costs rose too much, employers complained that insurers did not add value, and insurers responded with utilization management of, and discounts from, preferred providers with whom they contracted for services. As providers respond to managed care by organizing into larger delivery systems (multispecialty groups, IPAs, PHOs, physician practice management firms), payers may respond by trying to own the information systems that link providers to each other and to members.

Collen writes somewhat pessimistically in the Journal of the AMIA: "It will be increasingly clear that whoever owns the computer-based medical patient records, with their wealth of data about clinical processes and outcomes, controls patient care. Large insurer-owned, for-profit MCPs (managed care plans) will continue to expand their control over their contract physicians' clinical practice by exploiting clinical data."[22]

Whether insurers or medical groups are in control of clinical practice is largely a moot point if you believe that larger health care organizations of providers will emerge that take financial risk and obtain the information processing infrastructure to manage health care costs from payers. The health care organization will be both payer and provider, like the Kaiser organization and large group model HMOs are today. Information systems will be indispensable to the survival of these health care organizations. They will depend on the architecture of the Internet for their foundation and will link providers, payers, members, and patients into an electronic web for easy communication. The capital and systems expertise of payers will play an important role in helping the health care organization of the future succeed in the marketplace.

1. Relman, A. "Assessment and Accountability: The Third Revolution in Medical Care." *New England Journal of Medicine* 319(18):1220-2, Nov. 3, 1988.

2. Ellwood, P. "Shattuck Lecture-Outcomes Management. A Technology of Patient Experience." *New England Journal of Medicine* 318(23):1549-56, June 9, 1988.

3. "Data Minefields." *American Medical News,* Jan. 4, 1999.

4. "If Hospitals Do Data Mining, They Must Protect Patients." *American Medical News,* June 15/22, 1998.

5. *Columbia Dictionary of Quotations.* New York, N.Y.: Columbia University Press, 1995.

6. Needleman, J. *Money and the Meaning of Life.* New York, N.Y.: Currency Doubleday, 1991.

7. Wennberg, J. "Understanding Geographic Variations in Health Care Delivery," *New England Journal of Medicine* 340(1):52-3, Jan. 7, 1999.

8. Birkmeyer, J., and others. "Variation Profiles of Common Surgical Procedures." *Surgery* 124(5):917-23, Nov. 1998.

9. Wennberg, J., and others. "Practice Variations and the Challenge to Leadership." *Spine* 21(8):910-6, April 15, 1996.

10. Deming, W. *Out of the Crisis.* Cambridge, Mass.: MIT Press, 1986.

11. Juran, J. *Juran on Leadership for Quality: An Executive Handbook.* New York, N.Y.: Free Press, 1989.

12. Crosby, P. *Quality Is Free: The Art of Making Quality Certain.* New York, N.Y.: Mentor Books, 1992.

13. Berwick, D. *Curing Health Care: New Strategies for Quality Improvement.* San Francisco, Calif.: Jossey-Bass, 1990.

14. Eddy, D. *Clinical Decision Making, From Theory to Practice.* Sudbury, Mass.: Jones and Bartlett, 1996.

15. "Extreme Liposuction Is Exposing Patients to Unnecessary Risk." *Wall Street Journal,* Jan. 18, 1999, p. A1.

16. Brook, R. "Managed Care Is Not the Problem, Quality Is." *JAMA* 278(19):1612-4, Nov. 19, 1997.

17. Brook, R., and others. "Quality of Health Care. Part 2: Measuring Quality of Care." *New England Journal of Medicine* 335(13):966-70, Sept. 26, 1996.

18. Schuster, M., and others. "How Good Is the Quality of Health Care in the United States?" *Milbank Quarterly* 76(4):517-63, 509, 1998.

19. Froehlich, F., and others. "Performance of Panel-Based Criteria to Evaluate the Appropriateness of Colonoscopy: A Prospective Study." *Gastrointestinal Endoscopy* 48(2):128-36, Aug. 1998.

20. Vader, J., and others. "Appropriateness of Upper Gastrointestinal Endoscopy: Comparison of American and Swiss Criteria." *International Journal of Quality in Health Care* 9(2):87-92, April 1997.

21. Fuchs, V. *Economic Aspects of Health.* Chicago, Ill.: University of Chicago Press, 1982.

22. Collen, M. "A Vision of Health Care and Informatics in 2008." *Journal of the American Medical Informatics Association* 6(1):1-5, Jan.-Feb. 1999.

# Section II
## Expanding Horizons

# Chapter 10
## The Wonderful Evolution of Personal Computers

Here I am in late 1998, flying to Chicago, then on to Portland, and on my lap is my new IBM 770ED, with 128 megabytes of RAM, a 266 megahertz Pentium II microprocessor, 8.1 gigabytes hard drive, 100 megahertz Etheret LAN card, 14.1 SVGA graphics resolution screen, and DVD drive. I just replaced the now inadequate Compaq LTE5200 I wrote about in 1996 in the introduction to what was then this chapter. The Compaq could not handle the bloat of software in Office 97, IE4.0, Outlook 98. This currently amazing computer, with two docking stations, cost $3,000 less than the Compaq LTE5200 did in 1996.

Before I bought the Compaq computer, I used two computers for my work: a powerful desktop computer (Dell 133 MHz Pentium processor) to create courses and a notebook computer (IBM Thinkpad 75-MHz 80486 processor) to make presentations. The Thinkpad is adequate for making simple presentations, but not for the multimedia programs with high-resolution graphics (that now take up more than 100 megabytes of disk space) that I produce for the ACPE and for The Informatics Institute.

Having two computers was more of a nuisance than a convenience. Too frequently, I found myself copying files from one computer to another, to keep the most current version of an article, spreadsheet, or presentation on both machines. With files 100 MB in size, copying can take a long time, even with LapLink for Windows 95.

So, in mid-1996, I gave the Dell desktop and the IBM Thinkpad to my colleagues. I bought a Compaq LTE 5200 with an active matrix color monitor, 120-MHz Pentium processor, 1.35-gigabyte disk drive, a removable 4-speed CD-ROM drive, a 28,800-baud fax modem, a PCM-CIA 10BaseT ethernet adapter, and 75 megabytes of RAM. What a technological marvel this computer is! I recall that I said something similar, maybe even the same words, when I began using my first PC in 1983. This new computer fits effortlessly into a docking station in my office, which connects it to a local area network, an external keyboard and a monitor, and another hard disk drive for backups.

## My First Computer

I bought my first personal computer in the Mecca for PCs: Palo Alto, California, in the heart of Silicon Valley. I was studying business administration and health care economics at the Stanford Business School, after having finished my clinical training in internal medicine on the East Coast. My wonderful wife and I had our infant son with us, our first of four, and I wanted to spend less time in the computer laboratory and more time in our apartment.

So I considered personal computers. I selected the TI, an IBM-compatible system of sorts, in that it used an Intel 8088 processor, but with a proprietary graphics card from TI to give it better resolution than the CGA graphics of the IBM PC could produce. The Apple Macintosh had not been announced, and computers from Kaypro, Osborne, Radio Shack, DEC, and Apple did not seem as modern or reliable. But vendors had to rewrite part of their software to accommodate the TI graphics design. I assumed that, because the image was better, people would buy these computers preferentially and that the TI system would succeed in the marketplace.

Unfortunately, TI sold only a tiny proportion of the computers that IBM sold, and vendors lost interest in writing software for the TI graphics standard. In fact, TI abandoned its standard in favor of the IBM design within two years. Still, while I had it in business school I thoroughly enjoyed it. The interface was simple: primitive DOS from Microsoft, modified and supported by TI. The computer had a screen with 320 by 200 resolution, I believe; no hard disk drive (I added one later); 128K of RAM; and a 14-inch color monitor.

By today's standards, the PC was large and heavy. With it and Microsoft Multiplan, I could do all the spreadsheet analyses I had done with a DEC minicomputer in the data center at Stanford. I could do my work when I wanted to do it, at home, close to my wife and son, so we could walk to dinner at a small Mexican restaurant we loved and return to our apartment for me to continue my homework late into the evening. If I'd had a portable like the one I am using now, I would have carried it with me on my bicycle to the VA hospital in Palo Alto, where I moonlighted in the emergency department most weekends to pay my way through business school. Compaq, creator of the first successful IBM-compatible portables, did not yet exist.

After I graduated, I took the TI with me to Lakeland, Florida, where I became Medical Director of the Watson Clinic. I used it for two more years, but grew concerned that vendors were not writing new versions of their software for it. I thought I needed a portable computer, because I was beginning to travel to conferences and wanted to take work with me. I can type faster than I can write by hand, and almost faster than I can dictate, so a portable computer with word processing software would have been a godsend for me.

As an aside, the most important course I can recall taking in high school was typing. Far more than any single course in chemistry, English, geography, Spanish, history or mathematics, my course in typing has influenced my life in many beneficial ways. I have never been afraid of computers or their keyboards. And computers are much more appealing than the manual typewriter on which I practiced my lessons in class and at home.

I bought the TI Portable Pro, with the same architecture and processor as the original TI Pro, but packaged in a luggable computer weighing about 40 pounds, with a small 6-inch color monitor. It was only portable relative to the heavy TI Professional on my desktop. With no portables any lighter, I thought it was a marvel, and used it for the last year I worked at the Watson Clinic.

So, I used the same first-generation PC design for three years in a desktop and about one year in a portable. I added a little bit more RAM, eventually totaling 764K in a desktop that used an operating system that could not address more than 640K. That first generation lasted longer than any other. The pace of change in PCs began to accelerate in the late 1980s and continues to do so, and I began upgrading more frequently.

## My Next Computer

When Lotus 123 was released without a version for the TI Professional, I bought a TI Business Pro, which was compatible with the IBM PC AT, meaning it had the next generation of Intel microprocessor—the 80286. Contained in its massive tower case were a 40-megabyte hard disk, 2 MB of RAM, an EGA video card, and a 15-inch color monitor. It could run the newest version of Lotus 123. That baby was fantastic, but heavy as the dickens. Not portable by any means.

I was using early versions of WordPerfect for word processing and Lotus 123 for spreadsheet work. For database storage, I used dBASE a little. The interface for all those packages was based on text. With the EGA card, some simple graphics were possible, and I was comfortably mainstream, no longer envying IBM PC owners who, when I used the original TI Professional, had access to more software than I did. The Apple Macintosh had been available for several years by then, but, because of its small black-and-white screen and underpowered design, I chose to stay with the IBM standard. When I moved to Washington, D.C., in 1986 to join an HMO development firm, I sold the TI Portable Pro and took the TI Business Pro, with its larger hard disk space (40 MB), ample RAM memory (2 MB), and fast processor (80286), with me.

## Then I Moved to Compaq

I was traveling more than ever. When Compaq announced its second generation of portable PCs, the Portable II, with an 8-inch green monochrome screen, a 20-MB hard drive, 1 MB of RAM, and an 80286 Intel processor at about 4-MHz clock speed, I bought it. Back then, less than twelve years ago, the public would have had no way of knowing whether 4-MHz clock speed was good or not. Nowadays, even my eight- year-old son knows that a 233-MHz Pentium is middling fast, and a 400-MHz Pentium II processor is state-of-the-art.

Personal computers with multiple Pentium II processors are now available with clock speeds of 300-400 MHz, capable of 400+ million instructions per second. When the Portable II was first introduced, computer journals, including *Byte* magazine, featured photographs of Rod Canion, then the CEO of Compaq, holding it aloft with one arm, something most people could not do with most portables. The speed of its processor had little or nothing to do with its success. Its light weight won over converts. It weighed only about 20 pounds.

I loved that Compaq Portable II. I installed another 1 MB of RAM and a 40-MB hard disk card in one of the two expansion slots. In the other ISA slot, I put a sound card. The Hardcard cost at least $500 for 40 MB of disk storage, and so did the 1 MB of RAM. Now eight gigabytes of disk storage cost $300 and 1 megabyte of RAM sells for less than $5. I bought my first copy of Microsoft Windows, version 1.something, and suffered all the problems that you have heard about. I also loaded DesqView, a text-based interface, and sometimes used one, sometimes the other, to load my text-based applications from WordPerfect and Lotus.

Back then, Windows was not a user interface as much as it was a cool way to launch DOS applications. It crashed a lot or locked up the computer, and it was slow. I liked some of the utilities that came with it, especially the calculator. Most of the time, I preferred DesqView. I carried that computer to meetings in Minnesota, where we had started an HMO, to North Carolina and Virginia, where we were trying to start them, and to conferences. Even though by today's standards that little computer is very heavy and slow, I still have a great fondness for it.

Late in 1995 I gave it to my sons' school, and one of the teachers uses it for word processing and DOS-based games. Newer versions of Windows will not run on it, so its current owner uses a simple text interface to launch programs, one at a time. But I used that Portable II as my only computer for about two years, and as a computer for our home for about six years, although we added more modern computers to our inventory along the way. My fondness for Compaq computers derives from that gem of a Portable II.

### Along Came Intel

In 1987, along came Intel's first 32-bit microprocessor, the 80386, and Compaq beat IBM to the market with a desktop computer containing it called the Deskpro 386. I bought one immediately. It had a 40-megabyte hard drive, an EGA video card, a 15-inch external color monitor, and about 2 MB of RAM and processed at about 8 MHz. I used it at work for modeling business plans on Lotus 123, and for word processing. Boy, was it fast, and it could run Windows more reliably, addressing more memory, than the Portable II could.

This was the second time that I found myself using a desktop computer at work and a portable at home that I would take with me on trips. The richness of the computing power around me offset the inconvenience of swapping files. At least back then I could copy all the files I worked with to a single floppy disk. I used text-based DOS applications that took up little memory to store. That was about to change, as I began to dabble with early versions of Microsoft Windows.

I read favorable reviews about Microsoft software designed for Windows, such as Excel and Word. But they were slower than my DOS applications. I continued to use Windows for my interface, although I loaded DesqView occasionally. Then, in late 1987, I heard about Framework, an integrated package of software from Ashton-Tate with features for word processing, spreadsheets, and database. I used it for several months, but decided it had no benefits over WordPerfect, Lotus 123, and dBASE.

### Time for Another Compaq

Less than two years passed, and, in 1989, I bought a Compaq Portable III, with a faster 80386 processor than I had in my Deskpro 386. It was also lighter than the Portable II. So, now I hoped I'd have one computer for all my work. The Portable III used a novel lunch box design with a moveable amber flat panel screen. It had room for two full-sized ISA interface cards, an internal hard disk with about 80 MB of storage, and room for about 4 MB of RAM.

*The Wonderful Evolution of Personal Computers* 65

I usually upgrade computers because they have become too slow or restricted in RAM or hard disk space. Back then, reliable disk compression utilities were not available. Compaq and IBM started competing head-to-head in the market for portable computers, bringing out substantially more appealing designs about every 12 to 18 months. It was Windows that fueled my insatiable thirst for faster processors, larger hard disk drives, and more RAM memory in lighter, more portable cases. I was entering a period in which I switched PCs almost every year.

**The IBM Portable Era**
In 1990, the IBM Portable, based on a 33-MHz 80486 processor, was introduced. This new processor got a lot of attention. It had a 32-bit internal and external data path, so it moved data to the computer's circuitry more quickly than the 80386 and had faster processing speeds. This portable had more space for modem, video, and sound. Its marvelous flat monochrome orange screen, ample room for expansion cards and hard disk, and great keyboard converted me. It had a peculiar Microchannel bus, so I bought an expensive SoundBlaster card that I could not use in any other computer, but it produced great sound.

I had entered my IBM portable period. My first presentations for the American College of Physician Executives were made using Microsoft PowerPoint and the IBM Portable. I delivered my message with computer-driven slides. Even though my arm stretched whenever I carried its 30+ pounds, I took it everywhere happily. It did not have a battery, but I preferred a fast computer with AC power rather than a smaller notebook with a monochrome screen and slower processor. It had an early 80486 processor, about 8 MB of RAM, and a 400-MB hard disk that filled up quickly when I began to use Microsoft applications running under Windows.

I used that luggable portable for about a year, until IBM released its first 80486 notebook, an early Thinkpad, with a color monitor, full-sized keyboard and sufficient RAM and hard disk memory to run Windows 2.whatever. It ran on battery power, but they were nickel cadmium batteries that did not last long (less than one hour) and quickly lost their full charge due to an annoying memory effect. It was a large notebook, but much smaller and lighter than the IBM Portable.

**Back to Compaq**
I used the IBM Thinkpad briefly, perhaps nine months, until, in 1991, Compaq released the Portable 486c, a lunch box with a 66-MHz 80486 processor, gorgeous flat panel color monitor, 500-MB hard drive and room for two full length ISA cards. It did not use batteries, but I gave up the ability to use it on airplanes to have a better screen image, larger hard disk drive, and room for internal network and sound cards. The PCMCIA cards (about the size of credit cards) for notebooks had not arrived on the scene yet, but they would eventually eliminate the market for luggable computers with room for full-sized ISA expansion cards.

I switched to the Compaq Portable 486c, although it was slightly heavier than the IBM notebook, because it had a better color monitor, more RAM with which to run Windows 3.0, a larger hard disk drive, and room for a sound card I found indispensable (for games). It weighed about 15 pounds. It ran Windows 3.0 and Microsoft Office applications well, with a 500-MB hard disk and 16 MB of RAM.

Then Compaq began using PCMCIA cards and produced a notebook computer, the Contura, with a 50-MHz 80486, a great color monitor, and a 340-MB hard disk. It weighed less than 8 pounds. Who would not give up a heavier lunch-box-sized luggable for a color screen on a much lighter, faster computer with just as much disk space and RAM?

**Another IBM**
I used the Contura for less than a year, because I was making presentations with Microsoft PowerPoint and wanted as much RAM, as large a hard disk, and as fast a processor as possible. So I switched back to IBM when its fast Thinkpads (Thinkpad 755c) with 75-MHz 80486 processors and state-of-the-art pointing devices came out. That machine holds a total of 32 MB of RAM and has a 500-MB hard disk drive, which I compressed with the DoubleSpace utility from Microsoft.

**Back to Compaq**
I started using the IBM computer in fall 1994 and stopped using it in 1996 when I got a Compaq LTE 5200 with the extraordinary features I mentioned above. By the way, with Drvspace, I had nearly 1 gigabyte of disk storage on the IBM Thinkpad, but it would not carry all the files I needed. The LTE 5200 I started using in March 1996 had a 1.35 gigabyte hard disk drive. I compressed it with Drvspace from Windows 95 for more than 2 gigabytes of disk storage. At first, after loading all my software, I had about 700 megabytes free. Within six months, I had deleted Drvspace because of data corruption problems and added a second hard drive in place of the floppy drive, for another 1.3 gigabytes.

The cost for a top-of-the-line notebook computer, fully loaded with RAM and hard disk storage and the fastest-available modem, has remained at about $7,000 for the past five years, while the features that this amount of money will buy have improved dramatically. In 1992, $7,000 would buy a 33-MHz 80486 processor, 400 MB of disk space, perhaps a maximum of 16 MB of RAM memory, and a 9,600 baud modem. In 1996, that money bought a 120-MHz Pentium processor (about 8 times faster in instructions per second), at least 40 MB of RAM, a 1.3 gigabyte hard disk drive (three times the data storage capacity), a 28,800 baud modem, and an internal quad-speed CD-ROM drive. In 1998, $6,000 buys an IBM 770ED with 266 MHz Pentium II processor, 128 megabytes of RAM, 8.1 gigabyte hard disk, 14.1 inch LCD color monitor with 1024x768 resolution, 4 megabyte video RAM, and a DVD drive for 10 gigabyte disks.

Just a few years ago, state-of-the-art monitors on portable computers were either dull color or monochrome amber. Now they are bright, vibrant, active matrix liquid crystal displays. The newest generation of portables arriving in stores now includes modular and interchangeable DVD-ROM drives and lithium ion batteries that deliver power for three to four hours each. These computers can send and receive NTSC television signals and present full-motion video on their screens. I didn't spend this much money to have a portable television set, but the fact that I have one inside my computer amazes me. This computer is ready for video conferencing! Just attach an inexpensive video camera to it, hook it up to a network, and I can send a video signal to another computer similarly equipped.

The IBM 266-MHz Thinkpad 770ED comes with a 14.1 inch diagonal screen. It holds up to 256 MB of RAM! It has stereo speakers, a Trackpoint III pointing device, and a DVD-ROM drive that swaps with a floppy drive, a ZIP drive, hard disk, or a battery. It accepts multiple PCMCIA cards for modems and network connectors. It is a fully capable desktop machine that is also portable, weighing about 9 pounds.

Now I have one computer for all my work, and use inexpensive docking stations to make connections to an external monitor at home and in the office. I have an ISDN connection to a LAN at home, so my PC connects to the Internet at 128 kbps. I don't know how long I'll wait before upgrading to something else, but that something else has not been announced, yet. I have preserved some of the limited capital of The Informatics Institute by having one machine with which I do all my work—in the office, at home, and on the road.

**Now My Sons Want Computers**
My two oldest sons are going off to school this fall and want computers. Their two younger brothers, who will stay at home for school, want computers, too. To rationalize the investment I expect I'll make in computing resources for the entire family over the next decade, I tell myself I'd rather have them learning to use computers than watching television. Then I think that they may want expensive portable computers so they can play video games and watch television wherever they go.

I frown and dismiss the thought. No, they'll use these expensive devices to do their homework wherever they want to study, take notes in class, and search the Internet for edifying information. I'm kidding myself. I dismiss that thought, too, and hope their mother and I have given them sufficiently good examples of the value of diligence and hard work to help them to use their time and our investment capital wisely. I thoroughly enjoy, and take full advantage of, notebook computers. I hope they do, too. Will I allow them to upgrade to new notebook computers every 12 to 18 months? I shudder at the thought.

# Chapter 11
## Linking Elements of System

Five years ago, when a health care community began to consider seriously how its members would implement an electronic communication network between workstations in all the locations of care, there were few options. Three proprietary firms were active in the business of bringing electronic data interchange to physician's offices: Integrated Medical Systems (IMS), a subsidiary of Eli Lilly; Health Communication Systems (HCS), a subsidiary of Blue Cross of Virginia; and Ameritech Health Connections, a subsidiary of the midwestern telephone company Ameritech.

These firms—and they now have other competitors too numerous to mention—license software for a communications hub and server to support messaging for electronic mail between participating providers, route laboratory and radiology results from regional laboratories and hospitals to providers, and verify eligibility and benefits with payers. They also license software for client workstations that permit them to interact with data on the server. The software is proprietary. Every copy installed costs the sponsoring health care provider money. Each workstation needs to be set up, and any interference with other business applications on any physician's or hospital workstation must be corrected. A community health information network (CHIN) linking hospitals and clinicians can amount to millions of dollars in licensing fees to the vendor, hardware costs for the communications devices and servers, and expertise to install the software on every computer on the network and train providers' staffs to use the network.

Is there a more economical architecture for a community health information network than the proprietary designs of IMS, Ameritech, HCS, and others? Today, the alternative is an extended intranet. Using World Wide Web (WWW) browser software, as well as servers that adhere to the WWW standards, an intranet is a private network, usually a local-area network inside a single office suite or building or a wide-area network linking various sites of a business. Until recently, most private corporate networks were isolated from public networks such as the Internet. Now, the World Wide Web has become so enticing to users that corporations have begun to modify their networks to allow any workstations on them to communicate outside of the private network, through firewall computers and digital telephone connections, to Internet access providers and the Internet.

As the popularity of the Internet's World Wide Web exploded in 1994 and 1995, corporations began adopting the browser software called Mosaic (and its derivatives) for their networks because the same software could be used to "surf" the Internet. Because intranets are easier to maintain and less expensive, they are replacing the more expensive "groupware" applications based on client-server architectures that corporations installed over the past five years. These intranets are based on widely available technologies designed for the Internet, not on proprietary software designed for a relatively few customers.

The World Wide Web standards on which an intranet is based become a kind of inexpensive interface gateway, allowing any corporate application to communicate electronically with any other corporate application. On an intranet, the interface to the patient accounting system will resemble the interface to the order-entry, results-reporting system, which will resemble the interface to the laboratory system and the computer-based patient record.

The features of these various points of access to corporate data in different computer systems are produced by HTML (hypertext mark-up language) and XML (extended mark-up language), which are common to most applications on the World Wide Web. Now, with a huge installed base of Web users, the Web browser software vendors (Netscape, Microsoft, Spry, and others) can invest hundreds of millions of dollars improving their products but still charge minimal fees to license them to individuals.

These economies of scale dictate that the World Wide Web standards become universal for health care communication networks and drive the proprietary designs out of business. I predict that, in the next few years, every physician will choose to connect his or her office to a community health information network based on the World Wide Web standards. Patients will communicate by intranets and the World Wide Web. In parts of the United States, nearly 60 percent of people have Internet addresses at work, at home (through CompuServe, Prodigy, America Online, and Microsoft Network), or at both sites. As the public adopts the World Wide Web for electronic communication and the Internet for electronic mail, providers will have all the more reason to adopt Internet standards for their office practice networks and the regional communication networks they share.

If they adopt the ubiquitous standards of the World Wide Web, physicians will be able to communicate electronically with many of their patients, without having to install and maintain expensive proprietary software on patients' and health plan members' computers. Then the networks truly will be community health information networks—patients and health plan members will have the same benefits of continuing education on health promotion and disease prevention and secure transmission of laboratory results and e-mail that their physicians use.

Security is an important issue. The security features of major Web browsers will be much more robust than those of proprietary community health information networks, which have fewer customers and less capital for maintenance and modernization. VISA and MasterCard have agreed to a sophisticated security methodology to protect financial transactions over the World Wide Web. Those same features can be used to make clinical communications secure, even over public phone lines between physicians' homes and offices and through computers used by health plan members and patients.

*Linking Elements of System*

Organizations with communication networks integrated with their transaction systems and electronic medical records will be more effective in managing health care resources—and more attractive to employers and insurers for managed care contracting.

# Chapter 12

## The World Wide Web Is Coming Soon to an Organization Near You

The World Wide Web, a subset of the Internet, is coming soon to an integrated delivery system, hospital, group practice, health plan, IPA, PPO, PHO, or MSO near you. You will use it for patient care and public health and organizational management before you know it. It will replace the few proprietary community health information networks that exist now and will catalyze growth of electronic medical communications of all sorts between physicians, patients, facilities, payers, regulatory agencies, and members of the general public. It will allow you to videoconference with your colleagues, teleconfer with your patients, test yourself on new medical knowledge without visiting a testing center, and select a clinician for your new medical complaint from the comfort of your own personal computer.

Many experts argue that the Internet is the next paradigm shift in computing, the one after the personal computer. They predict the standards that define the Internet will accelerate the arrival of the information superhighway as a ubiquitous, standardized computing platform. It is already capable of transforming many of the ways in which physicians practice medicine. It is changing the ways in which our patients learn about their conditions, how they care for themselves, how they learn to avoid ailments, and how they reach medical attention when they need it.

The World Wide Web (WWW), sooner than any of us would have predicted two years ago, has defined, and is defined by, a set of standards and technologies that allow us to construct true community health information networks, linking electronically all members of the community involved with our health care services. The WWW provides the technical design necessary for standardized, vendor-independent, computer-based patient records to flourish.

So forget all that you have heard about community health information networks that require your organization to contract with a vendor of proprietary software, supply a copy of that software to every potential user of the network, and support that software with staff. Consider instead what a global open standard network can do for you, your patients, your organization, and your community. And the same standards that make global, ubiquitous computing possible allow organizations to place Internet-standard network servers (computers themselves) with information proprietary to those organizations on corporate local and wide-area networks to make that information available to employees in electronic form—such as documents for personnel policies and operational instructions and directories of employees, with photographs, graphics, sound, and video clips of them. The WWW and intranets using WWW software share standards for digital networking that may undermine the market value of many proprietary systems, because they establish a vendor-independent, personal computer-based platform for computing, networking, and teleconferencing.

The World Wide Web of the Internet is available to anyone who has an account with a computer communication services firm or with an Internet access provider. An intranet uses the same communication protocols, standards, and technology that define the World Wide Web. Intranets are growing as corporations discover that they can purchase and install World Wide Web servers that give their employees many of the benefits of multimedia documents, interactive forms, accessible databases, and other features of the most advanced public Internet sites. They can do so at far less cost than they might otherwise spend to maintain proprietary document management systems on their networks. And the latter have fewer, and more slowly developing, features than those available for the Internet. The computing standards that define the Internet are becoming more advanced, more replete with features, and more exciting than those of proprietary vendors' networking products, because there are so many vendors writing for the Internet and many fewer writing for proprietary systems.

Internet standards have existed for 30 years. The basic Internet standards for communicating data were developed for the Department of Defense. The standards, Transmission Control Protocol (TCP) and Internet Protocol (IP), together make up the TCP/IP protocol stack that allows computers to break up files to be sent electronically between them into packets of data. Each packet is given specific bits that identify the computer that created them, the computer that is to receive them, and the total number of packets that must move from the sending machine to the receiving machine before all the parts of the digital file are received at the receiving machine.

TCP/IP protocols also include rules that the computers follow to keep track of which packets they have received and which they have not. If packets are lost in transit because of some failure of the network, the recipient computer signals the sending computer to resend specific packets that did not arrive. The recipient computer knows which packets it lacks because each packet contains instructions on how many packets there are and in what order they must be received at the recipient computer for it to have all the data that make up a particular file. The file is useless to the recipient computer until all the packets are received and reassembled. The Internet Protocol established the conventions for addressing computers on the Internet so that sending, receiving, and intermediate transmitting computers know where to send packets as they produce, transmit, and receive them.

This design puts the intelligence for routing messages into the messages themselves and obviates the need for a central computer to decide how to move data from one computer to another. Without the need for a master switch, the entire network is far less vulnerable to unintentional, or intentional, failure. In fact, the network was designed with routing instructions embedded in the packets to make the network far less susceptible to damage from nuclear attack than it would have been had it contained a central switching site. TCP/IP protocols were designed in the 1960s, at the height of the cold war, to protect communication of data electronically among computers in government facilities, universities, and defense contractors that were used by the Department of Defense for research purposes.

So why does this design lend itself to corporate and community computing, and why has use of these Internet standards exploded in popularity with the general public? Use of the Internet was limited to communication of e-mail messages and digital computer files between universities, government agencies, and a few private firms for all but the last five of the past 40 years, with the general public and commercial firms paying little attention. Then, in 1992, researchers at the European Laboratory for Research Physics in Cern, Switzerland, created a set of software protocols for moving text, images, and all other digital files over the Internet with a graphical user interface on client workstations. They called the subset of computers (clients and servers) on the Internet using those protocols the World Wide Web.

In September 1993, programmers at the University of Illinois released the first browser software for the World Wide Web for IBM-compatible personal computers running Microsoft Windows. Called Mosaic, it was free of charge for anyone who knew how to access the server on which the binary files for it were stored. Interest in Mosaic quickly grew huge. Graduate and undergraduate students at universities all over the world notified each other by e-mail messages about its location and copied the files for Mosaic to their servers to make more copies of Mosaic available on the Internet more quickly. Interest and use of Mosaic, and the World Wide Web, grew exponentially. People now had a relatively easy way to access multimedia documents on computers all over the world by simply pointing and clicking on text names in other documents on the WWW.

The principle beauty of the World Wide Web, and of the browser software Mosaic, is that addresses of computers on the WWW are in natural language; their arcane numeric computer addresses are hidden from view. Users simply click on the words Stanford University, embedded in text on the home page (an introductory multimedia document on the WWW) of another computer on the Internet to visit the home page of Stanford University. In that document may be a reference to a document on a computer in Japan. By simply clicking on the name of the document in Japan, the WWW handles the complex routing instructions to download that document off a server in Japan to the user's workstation using the Mosaic browser, no matter where the user's computer is located.

The ease of surfing the Internet is staggering, compared to the mystery of programming logic and the hassles of text menus that preceded the point-and-click interface of the WWW. Operators of most of the servers on the Internet are converting their server software to make them compatible with WWW standards so they can contribute their information to anyone on the WWW inclined to visit their sites with browser software compatible with client WWW protocols.

The World Wide Web technology of the Internet is being adopted rapidly within corporations to create intranets for their internal communications. Corporations can maintain the security benefits of their own private local and wide-area networks and still enjoy the benefits of rapidly emerging new products and services for intraorganizational, client/server computing based on open standards. Use of these standards for electronic computing may grow from 35 million people today to more than 200 million people in three years. With such a huge market for shared standards, suppliers of products and services will produce more exciting applications for users than any one firm controlling a proprietary set of standards ever could produce.

What does all this mean for health care services and your own organization? I see two areas of enormous opportunity for health care organizations that choose to use the Internet standards for electronic communications:

- Internal organizational communication, including interactive and secure communications.
- External organizational communication with members of the community, including participating physicians, other allied providers, health plan members, patients, and the general public.

Without the Internet, organizations may communicate by proprietary means internally and with allied external entities to whom the organization has given the software, but they will be hard pressed to distribute and support the software to permit allied providers, health plan members, and the general public to communicate with them electronically.

What could a health care corporation do with an intranet? It could disseminate manuals and documentation of all sorts to its stakeholders. Placing most corporate policy manuals, telephone directories, schedules of events, electronic mail directories, corporate histories, and all documents usually made public on the corporate intranet allows any employee with an Internet browser on his or her personal computer, and a password to the system, to access them. The corporation increases the number of persons with legitimate needs who can see and peruse the documents, while reducing substantially the costs of production and distribution in paper. They can always be kept current in electronic form without the need to print thousands of new copies for each new edition.

In the long run, far more important to corporations are the new functions for creation of data entry forms in client WWW browsers. Employees could enter data into transaction systems and launch search routines in corporate transaction systems to find data important to their work. Physicians can search medical records using their WWW software, after entering through a security checkpoint, and read, but not write, to the databases into which they make inquiry. Health plan members and patients can access databases about services, including classes, available through the health care organization. They could check simple rule-based guidance systems for symptoms or questions about procedures and treatments they may have and gain access to answers to their questions when their providers are not available to them.

The ACPE debuted its presence on the World Wide Web at its Future Forum in La Jolla, California, at the end of January 1996. Anyone can complete a form to register for a course or purchase a publication from the ACPE by typing information ACPE needs to complete a transaction into a form made available by hypertext link on the bottom of every page describing publications or seminars.

Browser software can be used in many health care and medical settings to allow many different stakeholders of health care organizations—employees, affiliated physicians, or members of the general public—to have access to documents placed on a WWW server. For instance, patients can complete health risk assessments or functional status and satisfaction surveys on-line from their homes or offices, having been alerted by electronic mail when they are due to complete them. A forms interface allows members of the public, or health plan members, to enter their complaints into an expert system that can give them counsel on the best means to manage their conditions. This reduces the cost of nurses, clerks, and physicians answering the telephone and trying to deal with such questions, without the benefit of standardized answers in front of them.

Some patients and health plan members enjoy searching a database on participating physicians to see pictures, read text descriptions, and even hear statements from physicians describing themselves and the types of patients they serve best, all as a way to help patients or health plan members select physicians for their care. Physicians can send laboratory results to patients who want to receive such messages by electronic mail. Some patients have security clearance to dial in and check on the results of their laboratory studies directly, which is a convenience for patients on coumadin, diabetics, and those with chronic renal failure, all of whom need to be active in their daily care.

Physicians, or their staffs, find it very convenient to connect to an Internet server to check on the benefits and eligibility of people who appear in their offices for treatment and to obtain lists of providers participating in specific health plans to whom they can make referrals. With standardized documents and forms already on the Internet server, the processes for obtaining prior approval for planned treatments and for sending requests for consultations to subspecialists are made much easier and faster. Patients scheduled for specific procedures, or preparing to take specific medications, can look up explanations of their ailments and instructions on preparation for procedures or other treatments on their health care organization's WWW server. Office staffs can print such documents, saving their physicians time in reciting what the documents spell out in print. The forms function can be used to allow providers to submit claims in standard HCFA 1500 format on the WWW server and, with sufficient security protection, even schedule hospital facilities for procedures on patients and order medications with an on-line signature. Participating pharmacies receive prescription orders from physicians' offices in the same way.

Anyone familiar with community health information networks (CHINs) has probably already thought that all the functions mentioned above, and more, can be performed on proprietary networks offered by a number of vendors. That is true, but the likelihood is very small that individual proprietary vendors will keep up the standards of their software to compete with those emerging for the WWW. Once an organization has adopted the standards of the WWW for communications between clients and servers, it can concentrate its resources on enhancing the functions it puts on those servers. It can also avoid the costs of maintaining and enhancing networking technologies for a relatively small group of people, compared to the entire world of users of WWW standards.

This is an exciting time to be practicing medicine and managing health care organizations. If you are not already doing so, we predict with utmost confidence that you and your organization will choose to "surf the net" much sooner than you would have predicted before you read this chapter.

# Chapter 13

## Surfing the Web

The Web is intoxicating. The ability to find useful information quickly from computers all over the world astonishes me. Recently, I called Directory Assistance to find the telephone number for a private school that my wife and I were interested in for our children. I knew the school's name, suburb, and the street. The operator scoured the directory assistance database, tried neighboring communities and various spellings to no avail and concluded that the school must not have a telephone number. She said that if the number had been unlisted, she would have been able to tell me so. This school is 50 years old and has more than 300 students. I doubted it had no telephone number.

My computer was on. I launched Internet Explorer via modem, searched the Web for the school using Alta Vista, without using street, country, or any other identifying information. In less than three seconds, up popped a list of about 20 documents with the name of the school included. The first document was a listing of the names and addresses of private elementary schools in Maryland. I scrolled down the page, and there was the school, address, telephone number, year it was founded, number of students, and grades offered. I had found the school's address and telephone number on the Web in seconds, searching a database many times larger than the one used by Directory Assistance. Score a victory for the Web.

### Search Services
The first haunts that physician executives should know how to find are the search services Alta Vista (http://www.altavista.com) and Yahoo! (http://www.yahoo.com). There are many other search utilities, including Lycos, HotBot, Web Crawler, Magellan, Excite, NetGuide Live, and InfoSeek. Each has its own strengths and weaknesses, but I have found everything I wanted to find on the Web with Alta Vista and Yahoo!

Alta Vista is a search engine developed at Digital Equipment Corporation. It searches every document on the Web and indexes every proper word. You can search Alta Vista by words or combinations of words using simple Boolean search concepts. You can use Advanced Search to identify documents in which one proper word or phrase is "near" another word or phrase. You can also search on exact phrases, including precise use of upper and lower case words. But Alta Vista imposes no discernible order on the documents that it retrieves.

For instance, you will find millions of documents with the words "heart" or "disease" in them. There will be fewer documents with the phrase "heart disease" in them, but still too many to review. If you search the National Library of Medicine, the articles will be in chronological order, or by language or author, because the NLM abstracts the articles in its knowledge base with many different key fields. With Alta Vista, you have little opportunity to search for specific types of documents. The value of Alta Vista is its comprehensive database of documents. The disadvantage is its relative lack of structure. It may list hundreds of documents with a few key words in them, some of use and most useless to you. Use Alta Vista to search for unusual phrases or names.

Yahoo! offers users a very different and complementary way to surf the Web. It employs human abstractors to visit Web sites and categorize them by the type of information they contain. If I had searched Yahoo!, I would have looked for documents involving private schools in Montgomery County, Maryland. With Alta Vista, I search for the proper names involved with what I want to find. If I want all the documents about a generic term, such as heart disease, I will find more sites on the Internet using Alta Vista; I will find a more organized set of sites where heart disease is a key concept with Yahoo!.

**National Library of Medicine**
There are many sources of medical knowledge on the Web, but, without a doubt, the most valuable place to search the medical knowledge base is Internet Grateful Med (http://igm.nlm.nih.gov/). This site implements the software for the National Library of Medicine's databases. You do not need to install client software on your computer. No longer do you need to install disks with Grateful Med search software that not long ago came in the mail for semiannual upgrades. Instead, because your Web browser gives you access to the functions of Internet Grateful Med, you enjoy the current version that is installed on the NLM server whenever you log into the site.

This is an example, by the way, of one of the potential benefits of converting transaction systems to the Web architecture, with the Java programming language to make them interactive. You can interact with any computer system modified to the Web design, without having to load client software. The Web browser becomes a universal client, greatly reducing one of the burdensome costs of the client-server design—having to maintain a standard version of client software on every computer for every application. Upgrading the Web browser software on client workstations is easy and can be performed automatically over the Web, the private Web-based network, or a corporate Intranet.

The National Library of Medicine also offers other sources of valuable information for clinicians, including the Visible Human project database (www.nlm.nih.gov/research/visible/visible_human.html), a massive effort to create a detailed three-dimensional archive of human anatomy, male and female. You can take two and three-dimensional virtual tours of human anatomy (www.crd.ge.com/esl/cgsp/projects/video/medical). The NLM also presents considerable details about the Unified Medical Language System (UMLS) at http://ftp.nlm.nih.gov/research/umls. The UMLS gives developers of computer-based patient records a structured methodology.

## Health Care Associations
Whenever two or more people meet to consider any topic of common interest, there will be an association. There are hundreds of associations devoted to medical topics. Some with the most informative Web pages include the **American Medical Association** (www.ama-assn.org/) and the **American College of Physician Executives** (www.acpe.org). At the former, you will find information about political activities in the house of medicine. In the latter, you will find the ACPE schedule of programs, membership information, a list of publications, and other material from or about the College, and members can take examinations online that lead to a Certificate of Medical Management.

**The American Hospital Association** has a site on the Web (www.aha.org). So does the American Nurses' Association (www.ana.org).

**The Voluntary Hospitals of America** has a site (www.vha.com) that describes its affiliated hospitals, programs, and services.

**The American Medical Women's Association** (more than 13,000 women) has a Web site (www.amwa-doc.org) worth visiting.

**The American College of Healthcare Executives** has a Web site for its constituency of administrators at www.ache.org. It describes the benefits of ACHE membership, including access publications and regional and national meetings.

**The Association of American Medical Colleges** has a colorful and informative site (http://www.aamc.org/).

One very ambitious site is that of **Columbia-HCA**, an association of hospitals owned by a parent corporation of the same name (http://www.columbia-hca.com). Columbia-HCA describes itself as "the nation's largest health care services provider." Columbia uses Macromedia Shockwave to present moving images and sound on its advanced Web site.

## Server Push Sites
PointCast network, developed by EDS Corporation and Reuters news service, is a server push technology, whereby software on your computer allows it to receive detailed information whenever the server pushes it at you. You can customize the software to indicate the stocks of the companies you follow, the weather of the regions that interest you, the news of the industries you read regularly, the professional teams that matter to you, and the stories from various news organizations you want to read. You can download the PointCast browser free of charge from www.pointcast.com for your PC. Advertising funds PointCast. I like the advertising; it is colorful and silent, less obtrusive than advertising on radio and television.

PointCast "pointcasts" tailored information to each client. It is not a broadcast, in that each client computer wants a unique mixture of the content on the PointCast server. The server pushes the information to your computer as soon as it is connected to the Internet and notifies the PointCast server that it wants an update of its information. If your computer is usually connected to the Internet through a corporate connection, PointCast will update it periodically, without your computer sending a request for an update. Server push technology, and the rapid maturation of the Web to commingle pull (you use a Web browser to request a document) and push (a server sends a message unsolicited to your computer), is described well in an article in the March 1997 issue of *Wired* magazine ("Kiss Your Browser Goodbye: The Radical Future of Media beyond the Web" by Kevin Kelly and Gary Wolf). With push and pull features maturing together, the Web becomes truly interactive, and far more useful and engaging than static Web pages.

Imagine pushing information to patients about how they can stay well, prepare for procedures, take medications properly, follow diets more closely, and select physicians for their children and themselves. Several health care sites have sprung up recently with push technologies at their core.

Intellihealth (www.intellihealth.com) is the result of a joint venture between U.S. Healthcare Systems, an aggressive HMO on the East Coast now owned by Aetna, and Johns Hopkins Health System. For free, you can agree to accept daily e-mail messages about various health care topics of interest to the general public. The messages are short, easy to read statements about incidence and prevalence of disease and about the results of new research. No experimental methods that have led to specific conclusions are presented, but contacts at Johns Hopkins often are mentioned in the notes. This free service has a more complete chargeable service sold to payers to help manage the demand of their health care beneficiaries. Now that health care providers are capitated, we are getting into the health education business in a much larger way to manage demand.

For the past 10 years, Ask-A-Nurse has competed with Dial Doctors to sign up hospitals for its doctor referral service. Ask-A-Nurse nurses followed "doctor-approved" protocols to triage patients to physicians' offices or emergency departments. Clerks working for Dial Doctors search extensive databases to identify physicians who might meet the needs of callers, by location, specialty, and insurance coverage, but they do not handle questions related to symptoms.

The parent companies of the two services merged to form Access Health (www.access-health.com), and the information content of their symptom-based triage protocols and their databases of physicians' characteristics are available over the Web, for a fee. Health plans contract with Access Health to manage demand of their beneficiaries, who are told to call a toll-free number before they select a physician or seek care in an urgent care center or emergency department. Access Health sells services for nearly 27 million covered lives and was publicly traded before HBOC acquired it in late 1998. While this site does not have push technology features yet, it undoubtedly will.

## Health Care Insurers and Health Plans

Many health care insurers have Web sites. The most sophisticated sites tend to be those of health plans with defined populations of people who may be more committed to their insurance because they get a delivery system as well as a means of financing health care services. Group Health Cooperative of Puget Sound, at www.ghc.org, shows the value of marketing favorable outcomes data. Group Health proudly displays its HEDIS statistics for the public to appreciate, especially all the benefits managers of corporations in the Pacific Northwest.

Harvard Pilgrim Health Care (www.harvardpilgrim.org) and Blue Cross and Blue Shield of Massachusetts (www.bcbsma.com) compete for business on the Web. Both insurers use their sites to allow beneficiaries to select physicians and learn how to take care of themselves and give information about their products and services.

Kaiser Permanente, the largest HMO in the United States, merged its Northern and Southern California regions at its site, www.kaiperm.org. It also provides a very visible display of information on food and health. Under Permanente Medicine, you can read about methods used in various Kaiser Permanente regions for reducing the hassle factor of receiving care. Here are some dramatic statistics from the site:

- "In Ohio, the concept is taken one step further in a pilot project. Through the use of a telephone pager system, referring physicians may ask specialists for advice and then directly access the specialists' schedules to make patient appointments. Currently, direct scheduling is taking place in cardiology, and, according to Walid Sidani, MD, Associate Medical Director of Operations in Ohio, eight departments will be on board this fall. Right now, specialists in nine departments carry consultation beepers."

- "Dr. Sidani has witnessed a 35 percent decrease in referrals into the urology department. Neurology has not only reduced visits by 50 percent, but has also cut the volume of electromyography (EMGs) by 80 percent due to more appropriate triage, as well as a decreased wait for tests from several weeks to just one week. Finally, the wait for a stress thallium test in cardiology has dropped from several months to 10 days."

The largest insurer of all, the Health Care Financing Administration (HCFA), has a site, at www.hcfa.gov, geared not to consumers of health care services at all, but rather to the communities of health services research and policy.

## Humor on the Net

There is a lot of humor on the Web—intentional and unintentional. Search the Web with a sense of humor. You can expect to find uniform resource locator (URL) codes that no longer work and sites whose name may be obvious to you, but not to the market. For instance, on the Web, www.ama.org is not the American Medical Association, but the American Marketing Association. The marketers beat the doctors to that coveted URL.

To find intentionally funny sites on the Web, search Yahoo! You'll find categories of sites for humor, tasteless humor, and political humor, among others. In fact, you'll find more than 75 categories of humor with more than 1,180 separate Web sites catalogued.

## Informatics Training Programs

The Informatics Institute's (TII) site, www.tii.ruffin.com, has detailed information on courses, the class schedule, and the faculty and a catapult site to other Web sites of interest to people in the health care industry.

The American Medical Informatics Association (AMIA) has a site, www.amia.org, where you can learn about the benefits of joining this association of thousands of physicians, nurses, pharmacists, managers, vendors, and consultants interested in computer applications in medicine.

The largest trade show on computers and medicine is organized by the Healthcare Information and Management Systems Society (HIMSS). Learn about HIMSS at www.himss.org.

There are many academic informatics research and training sites at medical centers around the United States. Some of the best known are at Duke (http://dmi-www.mc.duke.edu/), Stanford (http://camis.stanford.edu/), and the Center for Clinical Computing at Harvard University's Beth Israel Deaconess Medical Center (http://clinquery.bih.harvard.edu/). There are others, at Columbia and the University of Utah, for instance. The American Medical Informatics Association (AMIA) keeps a listing of training programs in informatics for physicians and nurses on its Web site at http://www.amia.org/lkedtr.html.

**Internet Companies**
There are so many interesting companies with a presence on the Internet! Some provide novel services via the Web or offer software for enlivening the Web pages. Some of my favorites are listed below.

The first is Bigger.Net, at www.bigger.net, the first firm to offer free, unlimited access to the Internet. You'll need to visit their Web page to learn the details, and which telephone numbers to dial with your modem to access its free Internet surfing service. The service receives its funds from advertising, but the ads are unobtrusive. This company moves the financing model of the Internet all the way to the financing model of television, in that the consumer pays for a terminal (television set in the case of the TV networks and a PC in the case of the Internet) and gets the programming for free. Advertisers pay for the cost of the programming and for the network.

At 1040ez.parsontech.com, a service of Parsons Technology, you can enter your data into an online tax return and send it electronically to the IRS, to get your refund sooner than you otherwise would. There is a fee, but only about $10, less than the $40 to $60 you will spend for tax preparation software.

BioMedNet (http://biomednet.com/) is a free service for which you will need an ID number and password to gain access to a vast world of biomedical information. BioMedNet earns income from advertisers and charges to members for searching medical literature for full text of articles. BioMedNet markets itself as the World Wide Club for the Biological and Medical Community. Members can join chats and discussions, post messages to each other, search a job exchange, and view full text articles from biomedical journals.

Everyone has probably discovered the CNN site on the Web, www.cnn.com, given the enormous advertising CNN and Turner Broadcasting have devoted to promoting it. This site is updated throughout the day, but it does not yet use push technologies. For the latest information, just refresh the screen to see if a new document has been posted. CNN Interactive creates the All Politics Web site at http://allpolitics.com/news/ for seriously addicted political groupies. It also offers CNNfn at http://cnnfn.com/index.html for financial news. CNN contributes content to the PointCast Web site.

CU-SeeMe at ftp://gated.cornell.edu/pub/video/html/Welcome.html is software developed at Cornell University that allows inexpensive video conferencing over the Internet, provided

*Surfing the Web*

both computers have Windows 95 or Windows 98 and video cameras, and both use CU-SeeMe software.

ESPNET Sportszone at http://espn.sportzone.com presents sports scores 24 hours a day. More sports scores, from more sports, than you could have imagined. I have not seen results of professional lava surfing or spear-dodging contests, but they can't be far off. You can play fantasy football and baseball at this site, too.

At HotMail, www.hotmail.com, you can sign up for a free account, and your e-mail will remain secure until you retrieve it. This is the least expensive way of giving e-mail addresses to every member of your family. HotMail receives revenue from advertisers, but the ads are not intrusive or troublesome. Microsoft owns HotMail

InterNIC, www.internic.net, is "a cooperative activity between the National Science Foundation, Network Solutions, Inc., and AT&T. AT&T supports Directory and Database Services. Network Solutions sponsors Registration Services, Support Services, and Net Scout Services," according to its Web site. InterNIC keeps track of domain names for the Internet and sells them on a first-come, first-served basis, with the exception that courts have ruled that people cannot grab names for which companies already have a copyright or trademark and hold the name hostage for ransom. I checked with InterNIC for Ruffin, and found that Ruffin.com was not taken. It is now, by my firm, Ruffin Informatics. You should claim your family name as a domain name before a cousin of yours gets it.

RealAudio is a venerable site. You can download for free the RealAudio software at www.realaudio.com to access radio stations over the Web. If you make a coast-to-coast trip, you won't be able to listen to your favorite radio station. But if that station collaborates with RealAudio and broadcasts on the Web, you can listen to that station anywhere on earth that you have a Web connection. Certainly, from a PC in any hotel in the United States. RealAudio works in concert with TimeCast, (www.timecast.com). RealAudio provides the software, and TimeCast schedules the broadcasts and keeps a listing of all the radio programs available over the Internet.

SportsLine USA (www.sportsline.com) allows you to follow live baseball games on the Net, with graphical displays of all the scores and statistics, as well as the location of players on the bases, in real time.

Everyone should know about SwitchBoard, an incredible service on the Web, also free, paid for by advertising, that allows you to look up the telephone number and address of any person or company in the U.S. The company acquires the electronic databases of telephone directories, and stores the data on an incredibly fast server. At www.switchboard.com, I typed my first and last names and discovered in less than two seconds the name, address, and telephone number of five other people named Marshall Ruffin. You can look up long-lost friends this way. It's amazing.

If you are interested in a vision of corporate education in the future, visit the Virtual Reality Institute, at www.vrinstitute.com. The purpose of this joint venture between EDS and Prosolvia Corporations is to develop technology for Web-based virtual reality training for employees of corporate clients.

## Hospitals and Hospital Systems

There are hundreds of hospitals and hospital systems with Web sites. Most are passive documents with little or no opportunity for interaction, except for the e-mail address of someone who will answer your questions. But a few are more ambitious and point us in the direction of using the Web to educate the public on a variety of topics related to health, wellness, preparing for procedures, managing ailments, and selecting providers. These are some of my favorite health care sites:

Catholic Healthcare West (www.chw.edu) uses graphics and text nicely to display the locations of its facilities and other affiliated organizations.

Columbia-HCA offers virtual reality tours of its facility, online chats with physicians, the results of quality and outcome studies, and online health manuals. Already there are multimedia educational programs about the human heart and about a child's tour of a Columbia Virtual Children's Hospital. It's a great site.

Duke University Medical Center has a simple educational site, www.mc.duke.edu. It also maintains a particularly useful site for those interested in standards for health care information systems, located at www.mcis.duke.edu/standards/guide.htm. Duke aptly uses the Tower of Babel as a symbol of the cacophony of incompatible standards that we all suffer with now.

There is an enormous listing of the Web pages of hundreds of hospitals in the U.S. at a commercial site that is free to search. Visit www.usaads.com/clients/hospital/hosp.htm and check out the hospitals and health systems in your community, state, or region that have a presence on the Web.

Mercy Health System, in Michigan and Iowa, uses the Web nicely to present its mission, key executives, and maps showing the locations of its facilities, www.mercyhealth.com.

## Miscellaneous

I keep a listing of about 45 interesting sites on the Web for which I don't have another category.

**Professional Football:** ABC's Monday Night Football maintains, even in the off season, an elaborate site where you can watch video clips and listen to the stirring sounds of the past season. Visit http://www.abcmnf.com/net30/index.html.

**Renaissance Art:** This online art gallery of oil paintings from the Renaissance allows you to copy absolutely gorgeous images from Raphael, Michaelangelo, Botticelli, and others. Visit the Addio Gallery (http://www.mcs.csuhayward.edu/~malek/Addio.html) at California State University, Hayward, for a feast of images and sounds. While you are perusing the art, soft music from the Renaissance will play through your speakers.

**Chevrolet** (www.chevrolet.com) uses the Web well to let you study its lineup of cars in ways more like visiting a show room than reading static brochures.

**The Computer Almanac,** listed on Microsoft's Web page as a "cool site" (http://www.cs.cmu.edu/afs/cs.cmu.edu/user/bam/www/numbers.html), lists details on trends in the computer industry, including numbers and types of computers sold and their various uses. This is a good site to visit if you are looking for latest information on the size and trends of the computer industry, or any part of it.

**Computer-Based Patient Records in Primary Care:** This unusual site is a listing of the titles and abstracts of 130 articles on computer-based patient records in primary care medicine. Robert B. Elson, MD, maintains the site. My hat is off to Dr. Elson for this valuable service. Visit http://www.nmsr.labmed.umn.edu/~relson/pubs/abs.html for the complete bibliography of articles.

**Health Insurance Portability and Accountability Act:** Read about this act that Congress passed into law in August 1996 (http://www.hostnet.org/hr3103.html). It will have profound implications for all providers and patients. The act calls for the creation of unique identification numbers for providers (physicians, physical therapists, pharmacies, and hospitals, among others) and patients to be used in all transactions, including claims and electronic communication for prior treatment authorization. You can download the entire contents of the legislation from ftp://ftp.loc.gov/pub/ thomas/c104/h3103.enr.txt.

**Bill Frist, MD,** a cardiovascular surgeon specializing in transplantation surgery, was the first U.S. Senator to have a Web page. He won the senate seat occupied by Senator Sasser from Tennessee in the 1994 elections. Frist uses the Internet frequently to reach his constituents and his staff. Visit him at http://www.senate.gov/~frist/directory.html and read about his voting record.

## Outcomes Management

The University of Texas School of Public Health maintains a Web page that lists hundreds of sites related to outcomes management. It is located at http://www.sph.uth.tmc.edu/WWW/RES/outcomes/outcomes.htm.

The California Consumer Health Scope site, www.healthscope.org, gives you a sense of where outcomes management programs are heading—in this case, provider profiling.

The Joint Commission on Accreditation of Healthcare Organizations (JCAHO) has a very ambitious program called ORYX to create a national dataset of outcomes data from hospitals, health plans, ambulatory care facilities, long-term care facilities, and integrated delivery systems. Read about ORYX and outcomes management at www.jcaho.org.

The National Committee on Quality Assurance (NCQA) developed HEDIS (Health Plan Employer Data and Information Set) to help employers evaluate the outcomes of health plans. The HEDIS data from health plans are now being published on the Web at www.ncqa.org as part of NCQA's Quality Compass initiative.

The Medical Outcomes Trust (http://www.outcomes-trust.org/home.htm) is a not-for-profit agency devoted to producing educational publications and conferences on the outcomes movement in health care. Its site is worth a visit.

## Publishers and Publications

Amazon Books is the world's largest bookstore of any type. It is a virtual store, available only on the Web, with more than 3 million book titles for sale. The site makes searching for, finding, selecting, and buying books easy and encrypts your credit card transaction. Visit www.amazon.com for a remarkable retail experience. You'll be tempted to buy more books than you can possibly read.

Most publishers of newspapers, magazines, and other periodicals have a presence on the Web where they put some or all of their content for your perusal. This is clearly a sign of the times. Reuters publishes on PointCast (www.pointcast.com). The *Washington Post* (www.washingtonpost.com), the *New York Times* (www.nytimes.com), and the *Chicago Tribune* (www.chicago.tribune.com) are on the Web. *Business Week* has a gorgeous site (http://www.businessweek.com/) full of fancy graphics. Even that colorful newspaper, *USA Today*, has an equally colorful Web site (www.usatoday.com).

Then we have the new publishing firms and the ones without a history of print publications. Ted Turner's CNN has several sites, including www.cnn.com for regular news, www.cnnfn.com for the new financial news service, and All Politics (http://allpolitics.com/index.html), a joint venture between CNN and *Time* magazine.

The NASDAQ stock exchange has an elaborate, colorful, graphical site where you can study with ease the performance of common stocks traded on the NASDAQ (http://www.nasdaq.com/).

Finally, MapQuest publishes, for free, detailed maps of the United States. You can search www.mapquest.com for a map of your community that shows your home. You can find out how to reach a destination.

**Telemedicine Sites**
Telemedicine, broadly defined, means the use of telecommunication technologies to deliver medical and health care services at a distance. One telemedicine company, Access Health (www.access-health.com), was already mentioned in the section on Server Push sites.

Without question, the best site on the Internet to learn about telemedicine is the Telemedicine Information Exchange, http://tie.telemed.org. The site receives its funding from the National Science Foundation, Pacific Telecom, and the Open Systems Foundation and exists on servers in Portland, Oregon. TIE lists thorough details on almost every major telemedicine project in the world, numbering more than 180 programs in 16 countries. You can read publications on telemedicine, search a library of comments by experts to frequently asked questions about the practical issues of starting a telemedicine program, and find links to most of the vendors of telemedicine equipment.

The Alaska Telemedicine Project is well described at http://www.telemedicine.alaska.edu/.

The Cyberspace Telemedical Office (http://www.telemedical.com/) is a proprietary example of telemedicine broadly defined. It offers knowledge bases for the public on how to care for common ailments; yellow pages of listings of providers by type and location; an opportunity to consult with a physician in an electronic "chat"; and a place to store your medical record, as you would record it, in digital form, with a password that only you can use. This service allows you to give a provider anywhere in the world linked to the Internet access to your medical record, as long as you provide your password.

The Department of Defense funds more research and development in telemedicine than any other agency of the federal government. You can visit the DoD Telemedicine Test Bed site (http://206.156.10.15) and sign up for regular e-mail messages describing its activities. You can see pictures of telemedicine equipment in MASH units in Bosnia. You can read about and see pictures of the Army's Mobile Medical Mentoring Vehicle (the M3V) that looks like a jeep with a satellite dish on top and video equipment inside. It is used for transmitting telemedicine images from the battlefield to MASH units and army hospitals at a distance from the casualties and is designed to support clinical triage decisions.

# Chapter 14
## Intranets Advance Medical Care

This chapter explores the technologies and benefits of intranets, including networks based on the standards of the Internet's World Wide Web (WWW). The Web is used by corporations and communities for semiprivate and private exchanges between members. Intranets will be advantageous to communities in many ways, including streamlining health care delivery. Medical groups, hospitals, payers, and patients will be able to share information electronically. Electronic networks linking providers, patients, and health plan members in these regional health care systems will be developed with the same technologies used to build the Web.

The Internet is coming to medical care in profoundly important ways, sooner than any of us would have predicted three years ago—in fact, sooner than most of us would have imagined even 12 months ago. These changes will not take place on the home pages of the Internet's World Wide Web. They will happen on intranets—corporate networks of group practices, hospitals, health plans, and PHOs that use Web standards but that are private.

And true community health information networks (CHINs) are coming soon. Community members will be linked—patients and potential patients, members of health plans and potential members—and will receive valuable services from access to CHINs spawned by providers and payers to make communication as convenient, efficient, and thorough as possible. Numerous networks will be offered in most metropolitan areas, each developed by an organization of providers or payers, to attract and retain customers.

There will be security provisions to keep private the information of patients, health plan members, and providers, while enabling the electronic exchange of data. Over the next five years, in many urban areas, networks will evolve to support multimedia communication, permit telemedicine practice, and make consultations with physicians convenient for patients. Who will pay for all these services? Clinicians and their health plans that use the technologies to competitive advantage.

Our society will enjoy an increase in the velocity and accuracy of medical diagnosis and treatment with these networks, and more focused and effective interventions to prevent illness. Providers and health plans will discover that CHINs will be indispensable tools for managing their limited health care resources and invaluable assets in their mission to wrest more customers from existing competitors. They will be as important as networks supporting automated teller machines are to banks and as networks linking travel agents to their flight schedules are to the airlines.

**Christopher's Story**

Imagine you have to treat a boy named Christopher. Christopher is 10 years old, bright and inquisitive, and inclined to make his own decisions. He complains of a bilateral, frontal headache at 4 p.m. on a Monday afternoon, as his mother is driving him home from school. She instructs him to take three chewable children's Tylenol tablets. He has taken them before and knows what they look like. In addition to the Tylenol tablets, his mother's purse also yields a sheet of Dimetapp Extentabs for adults, of which three are left. He reads the label and recalls that he has taken Dimetapp pills (for children) before and that they have made him feel better. Unbeknownst to his mother, he takes and ingests those three blue pills. They arrive home shortly afterward, and Christopher dives into his homework.

At 8:30 p.m., Christopher is lying in bed with a terrible headache, nauseated and vomiting. He has not eaten dinner and says he wants to rest. His mother attends to him, and asks him when his nausea started. He says shortly after he took those three blue pills. She gasps. She knows the Tylenol tablets are purple. She retrieves her purse. Christopher shows her the strip of Dimetapp tablets, from which he had taken the remaining three. His mother calls the pediatrician's office and then the poison control center. She also summons her husband from his study. Her husband is a physician, and she is a nurse.

The poison control center suggests they check Christopher's blood pressure, because Dimetapp Extentabs contain 75 mg of phenylpropanolamine, a decongestant that in large quantities can raise blood pressure, and 12 mg of brompheniramine, an antihistamine. Christopher weighs 70 pounds. He has taken about six times the recommended dose of each medication. The phenylpropanolamine may cause the most trouble. His parents check his blood pressure, which is 140/100, with a regular heart rate of 70.

The pediatrician is appraised of the circumstances. He calls the hospital emergency department and confers with poison control. Christopher's attendants choose to follow his blood pressure closely, but not to take him to the emergency department immediately. Because he took the medication four hours earlier and is already having dry heaves, they think the effects of ingested phenylpropanolamine may have peaked.

Every five minutes, Christopher's parents check his blood pressure, which rises to 160/120, with a regular heart rate of 65 over the next 10 minutes. His parents report this to the pediatrician and decide to take him to the emergency department. As they are preparing to leave, Christopher's mental status changes; he becomes stuporous. His parents race him to the emergency department where, moments after arrival, he suffers a series of focal seizures involving his left leg, followed within a minute or two by a generalized grand mal seizure.

The seizure is brief, less than 30 seconds, followed by normal respirations. Christopher never appears hypoxic. His heart rate is 60 and regular, his blood pressure 170/125. Emergency department staff members have an intravenous line in place and give him Valium IV, which stops the seizure activity and reduces his blood pressure. He is unresponsive and does not move his left side. Retinal examination is normal, without hemorrhages or papilledema. His pediatrician performs a literature search and learns that phenylpropanolamine in elevated doses may cause cardiac dysrhythmias and dystonic reactions, in addition to the hypertensive crisis Christopher has suffered.

Nevertheless, this is a story with a happy ending. Over the next 12 hours, Christopher recovers all of his neurological activity and is discharged after a normal CT brain scan—about 16 hours after his initial change in mental status and 20 hours after he ingested the wrong medication. His neurological deficits are considered to be transient, post-ictal paralyses (Todd's Paralysis). In two days, he returns to school with no apparent residual deficit.

He might not have been so lucky. His parents asked the right questions, determined his problem, measured his blood pressure, and got him to an emergency department before it was too late. Had his blood pressure continued to rise, had his parents not been able to check his blood pressure, had they told him to stay in bed and sleep his headache off, he could have sustained cerebral hemorrhages and permanent brain injury. He might have died.

Now imagine that the year is 2000, and Christopher is in bed with a headache, nauseated and vomiting. The community in which he lives has broadband telecommunication networks from competing, regional telephone and cable TV companies. His family does not include a father who is a physician or a mother who is a nurse. But, his family does subscribe to cable TV and uses a cable modem to obtain digital video signals for entertainment and videoconferencing.

They use the videoconferencing features of their entertainment and personal computer system, with a 36-inch monitor and 400 MHz Pentium II processor, to talk with family and friends. Their Gateway 2000 Destination system is three years old, but functions well. They have not used it to communicate with health care workers, but they will this evening.

Christopher's mother describes his severe bilateral headache and nausea to the pediatrician on call. The physician worries about a viral exanthem, perhaps a viral meningitis—she has seen several cases of it in the community recently. She asks to see and speak with Christopher. They walk to their living room to establish an encrypted videoconference over the community Intranet.

Their pediatrician moves to her workstation and reviews Christopher's uneventful medical history in his electronic record—to which she connects in seconds on her computer via the WWW, while she waits for the call establishing the videoconference, which occurs in a few minutes.

Christopher's mother has never participated in a home telemedicine session. She has never had to use the electronic blood pressure cuff and stethoscope their health plan sent them when they enrolled. These devices connect to a transducer that sends signals over the cable TV network. There is a small videocamera on top of the large screen entertainment monitor, allowing the pediatrician to see Christopher in his living room.

The pediatrician talks Christopher's mother through the proper use of the instruments, which takes about two minutes, and speaks to and observes Christopher. A large image of the pediatrician is on their home monitor, captured by an unobtrusive videocamera in the monitor of her workstation. She notices that Christopher obviously does not feel well, but seems to have normal mental status.

She asks him about his headache and when the nausea started. He says shortly after he took the medicine in his mother's purse for his headache. The pediatrician asks him to tell her what the pills looked like and he says they were blue and round. The pediatrician and Christopher's mother look at each other on their respective monitors. Chewable Tylenol are not blue, and they are not pills.

The physician asks Christopher's mother to retrieve her purse. She finds a sheet of Dimetapp Extentabs with three missing pills, and Christopher confirms he took them. He explains that he had taken Dimetapp before and they made him feel better, so he took them. His mother reminds him that he has taken children's Dimetapp before, but never Dimetapp for adults. The pediatrician says she wants to complete a brief physical examination of Christopher before she checks the poison control database.

His mother hooks up the blood pressure cuff, which also records heart rate, and the pediatrician sees on her screen a heart rate of 70 and regular and a blood pressure of 140/100. She is concerned. His parents (Christopher's father has joined them) hold the stethoscope where she instructs them to place it, as she watches Christopher. His lungs are normal. His heart is not. She hears a wide physiological splitting of the second heart sound, with a loud aortic component, but no third heart sound.

While that blood pressure, if transient, would probably not threaten Christopher, she knows, if it rises much further, he could be in serious trouble. She focuses the camera on his face and asks him a series of questions, all of which he answers well, though with tired and pained affect.

She asks his parents to stay in front of the entertainment center while she uses the community Intranet to revisit the poison control database and find information on the effects of a phenylpropanolamine overdose. The WWW site includes a spreadsheet, created as a Java applet, in which she enters the patient's age and weight, that he has normal renal and liver function, and that he took 225 mg of phenylpropanolamine four hours earlier.

The what-if analysis she performs indicates that the peak effect of the phenylpropanolamine is still probably more than one hour away and, if untreated, his blood pressure may rise to more than 180/130, with encephalopathy, seizures, and intracranial bleeding more likely. She decides the best course of action is to ask Christopher's parents to take him to the closest emergency department to treat his hypertension if his blood pressure rises any further or if there is a change in his mental status.

The pediatrician maximizes the window on her workstation. She asks Christopher how he feels. She notices that he seems slightly less alert and that his answers are more monosyllabic. She asks for another blood pressure reading and heart rate. His heart rate is 65 and regular and his blood pressure is 150/110.

With his blood pressure rising and his affect flattening, she decides there is no time to waste. She urges them to take him to the emergency department, where she will meet them. She signs off from the videoconference and makes a quick video call to the emergency department, informing the staff of Christopher's imminent arrival.

Six minutes later, Christopher and his parents arrive. He is walking, but tired and lethargic. His blood pressure is 160/120 and his HR is 60 and regular. Within five minutes, an intravenous line is in place, he is given sublingual nitrates and 1 mg of Valium IV. His blood pressure declines to 130/90, his heart rate increases to 75 beats per minute, he feels sleepy, and his headache diminishes. He stays for another four hours, then goes home with his parents, normotensive, with a normal neurological examination and minimum residual headache, for a well-deserved rest.

Christopher's real parents knew enough about medicine to ask the right questions and get him to an emergency department in time to prevent probable serious sequelae from his drug-induced hypertension and seizures. With the advent of videoconferencing and home telemedicine sessions, we hope more situations such as the one Christopher suffered can be avoided. Health care networks will offer parents the peace of mind of readily available videoconferencing from home, on-line poison control databases, and electronic medical records with password and encryption protection.

## Why Develop Intranets?

An Intranet is a corporate asset, not a public service. It is a network connecting the stakeholders of an organization, allowing users to share data with browsers designed for the WWW. It uses hypertext mark-up language (HTML) and virtual reality mark-up language (VRML) to create documents retrievable over the Intranet and JAVA application programming language to create small applications (applets) that make the intranet interactive. These networks adopt the browser and server software of the Web to bring multimedia information to corporate workstations using widely available technology.

Intranets are used to publish corporate newsletters and other periodicals, distribute policy manuals and instructions for operating equipment, maintain up-to-date directories of personnel and facilities, and give users access to news and discussion groups. The Intranet can serve as a standard data entry device to allow employees to enter their ID numbers and passwords for inquiries about their retirement plan account balance, or for clinicians to enter patient ID numbers and their own passwords to check on laboratory results and radiologists' interpretations of diagnostic studies. Corporations can take advantage of the enormously productive ferment in the communications industry and the improved software being designed for the Web. Corporations that use WWW standards on their private networks will not have to worry that they will only improve with the pace of a single vendor. Vendors may come and go, but the WWW standards will continue to mature at an astronomical rate.

In most developed countries, practically everyone will have an Internet address within the next few years. Each person will have at least one personal computer that can access the Web and know how to navigate it. The training costs for corporations that use those same standards for networking their computers will be far lower than the costs for those that use proprietary software unfamiliar to employees and other stakeholders with whom they want to share digital communication.

Designed as intranets, community health information networks will link the homes and offices of people in a given geographic area with health care plans and providers. Software must be familiar to the staff in physicians' offices and the general public to induce them to use the network. No health care organization is going to spend the resources needed to install proprietary software for its network in the homes of patients, potential patients, health plan members, and potential members. But all those groups will have access to any CHIN designed with WWW standard browser software, as long as they have passwords to the network itself. Passwords are much less expensive than copies of proprietary software to distribute to a large audience. For the latter, the health care organization must pay the developer as well as the additional costs of installation and training.

## How Health Care Stakeholders Benefit

Patients, health plan members, physicians, nurses, allied health professionals (physical and respiratory therapists, dieticians, psychologists, occupational therapists, radiology and laboratory technologists, and physicians' assistants, to name a few), administrators, family members of patients, pharmacists, regulators of the health care industry, suppliers to the industry, insurers, and communities that depend on health care providers all are important stakeholders. And each could benefit from Intranet technology.

## Members of Health Plans

***Explanation of covered benefits:*** Members want to learn about their health care benefits before they need to use them. They want to know how to select a primary care physician for each family member, if their plan requires that they declare one, and use him or her for guidance. Members know that many services will not be paid in full, or paid at all, unless they receive their primary care physician's approval to use them. Imagine that members could use the personal computer they use for balancing their checkbooks and calculating their taxes to check on their health care benefits electronically.

***Clerical and administrative reporting***: Most administrative offices of health plans are open from 9 a.m. to 5 p.m., Monday through Friday. When members are at home working on claims forms and family budgets, no one is available to answer their questions. Members could check on the status of claims they have submitted in the past three years, any time of the day or night, by entering their personal ID number and password. With that same computer, they could select a physician from a multimedia biography—complete with a photograph, a brief videotape describing his or her training and beliefs about practice, and availability to take new patients.

***Preventive medical services:*** Members want to know that their health plan will alert them when screening procedures are due (PAP smears, sigmoidoscopies, tetanus boosters, flu shots, mammograms). They want to know if they are at risk for preventable diseases and how to stop them from occurring. Members want to complete health risk assessments on the home page of their health plan using a PC and see their answers immediately—what specific steps to take to reduce their risk of common chronic ailments. The answers could be copied to the electronic mail file of the primary care physician and added to the member's medical record.

If each member were asked to complete an annual health risk assessment from the convenience of home via the Web, a file of valuable patient history would grow. The health plan would be on top of the member's risks and could advise on habits to remain healthy, relying on the electronic medical record and health risk assessments that the member helps to produce. Members prefer plans that emphasize preventive medicine and use modern information processing and knowledge bases to design specific health care regimens and help them avoid needing treatment.

## Patients

***Learning about what ails them:*** Each patient should learn as much about his or her ailment as possible, the life-style effect it is likely to have, the alternative treatments available, the costs, the possible unintended side-effects, and what to do to expedite recovery. The WWW provides opportunities for the patient to check on the results of recent diagnostic studies, read a layman's interpretation of the illness, look up recommended recipes, check the schedule of health education classes and support group meetings, and invite a new friend in a support group to lunch.

***Interactive learning engages patients and their families:*** Patients enjoy interactive learning online, such as completing health risk assessments and seeing the results immediately, interpreted in language they can understand. Today's fast Pentium computers with 31-inch monitors are available with the same capabilities as PCs. In addition, they have entertainment devices that attach to cable TV and modems to allow interactive electronic communication. The public will marvel at the merging of passive television viewing and computer gaming to produce interactive, educational, and entertaining video conferencing, with home entertainment equipment that doubles as a personal computer.

Ample evidence shows that a patient with a chronic illness who has family members who understand the disease and who can help provide care requires fewer medical resources, has fewer complications, and experiences less frequent acute exacerbation of the underlying condition. Just as telemedicine gives confidence to primary care physicians in rural locations who like to have a subspecialist confirm that they have made prudent choices for their patients, family members of patients with various cancers, neurological injury, acquired immune deficiency syndrome (AIDS), diabetes, and other chronic infections will benefit from periodic, brief electronic house calls by clinicians using telemedicine technologies.

## Physicians

***Telemedicine will facilitate acute care:*** Telemedicine consultations to physicians and allied health professionals will be common with teleconferencing equipment in the home. Many routine follow-up visits to physicians' offices and late evening visits to urgent care centers may be avoided with brief interactive videoconferences.

***Telemedicine aids primary care:*** The telemedicine program at the Medical College of Georgia has ample evidence that primary care physicians do well in their communities with occasional telemedicine consultation with subspecialists. More than 80 percent of the patients the primary care physicians would have sent to the academic medical center for a face-to-face consultation were successfully handled in their home communities with telemedicine. The patients do not need to travel, the primary care physicians learn how to manage unusual clinical situations, and the academic center builds a network of loyal community physicians who will transfer patients to it when the need arises.

The same digital networking technology that gives health plan members, patients, and their families access to multimedia documents about benefits and preventive health programs will permit videoconferencing from home with clinicians.

***Connect with all health plan members:*** Most providers don't know anything about the people they are not treating. Intranets offer them an opportunity to connect with members they ought to get to know and to inform them about how to seek care when they want it. The network helps keep people in touch, so to speak. It is a powerful means for the health care organization to manage the health and the ailments of its health plan members and patients and members whom the plan helps to avoid becoming patients.

The era of electronic medical care is already here. Physicians have computers in their homes and offices and know how to use them. They have access to the Web, using commonly available browsers from either CompuServe (using Spry's Air Mosaic); America Online, Prodigy, Microsoft (Internet Explorer); Netscape (Netscape); and other derivatives of Mosaic from any one of a number of smaller firms.

AT&T is forcing down the price for access, giving their long-distance customers five free hours on the Internet per month and everyone else a low fixed price for unlimited access. Cable TV companies—which already reach into tens of millions of homes and offices, including those of many physicians—offer Internet access through "cable modems" at data transfer rates much faster than those we can obtain with telephone modems.

While it may at first seem expensive to acquire the equipment and the knowledge to use the WWW, demographics of users show that every income group is well represented. Sales of personal computers capable of accessing the Web outnumbered television sets sold in the past three years, and the trend is estimated to continue. By the year 2000, most Americans will have PCs in their homes that resemble television sets.

Gateway 2000 has begun selling its Destination line of computers with fast Pentium processors, modems, and large hard disk and CD-ROM drives. Its monitor is 31 inches in diagonal size. It comes with a wireless, remote keyboard and controller and is ready for connections to standard coaxial cable TV. This device is a combination home computer and entertainment center. It is ready to attach to a camera to send video signals over a network, so it could be the sending and receiving station for teleconferencing.

This is the access point—physicians' own home pages on the WWW—for patients to learn how to care for themselves, about their health care benefits, and about preventive, diagnostic, and therapeutic services available from local hospitals, to participate in an electronic house call with a clinician at an urgent care center or emergency department. The advent of telemedicine into the home is nigh, and the Internet and WWW, or a local cable TV firm, will probably be first to carry the data in your community.

The equipment to access intranets for specific populations of patients and health plan members—with password protection to keep others out—is already in the homes and offices of most Americans, or will be shortly at very affordable prices. The era of electronic medical care and home health is upon us. Innovative physicians will be able to extend their preventive and therapeutic practices to more patients in more locations.

## Conclusion

Today, all information can be stored electronically on the World Wide Web or on a private intranet, making data available more quickly to more people. As a result of the efforts of literally tens of thousands of engineers, programmers, and systems analysts, we will not only make all documents available electronically, but we will make them interactive—an invaluable function that books and journals cannot offer.

With interactive multimedia information sources, our abilities to teach, learn, instruct, and inspire will grow considerably. Patients will learn more about what ails them and how to care for themselves from interactive Web sites than they could from health plan newsletters and brochures. Patients and physicians will confer over the Internet. Doctors will consult with other physicians interactively over the Internet or on the intranets of their delivery networks. And children like Christopher will be less likely to suffer hypertension and seizures from misadventures with the wrong medication.

# Chapter 15

# Health Insurance Portability and Accountability Act of 1996

While physician executives were busy establishing their roles in hospitals and health plans, Congress created legislation that, in time, will elevate clinical leaders into the limelight of every health care organization. Congress passed the Health Insurance Portability and Accountability Act in August 1996 and promptly asked a committee with a storied and venerable history, the National Committee on Vital and Health Statistics, to begin working on the regulations that will help providers, payers, and all members of the public adhere to the spirit of the law.

You can download a copy of the legislation from the Thomas legislation server at Congress. The file transfer protocol (ftp) address is ftp://ftp.loc.gov/pub/thomas/c104/h3103.enr.txt. Type that URL into a Web browser and text will appear on your screen. You can print all 150 pages or simply read and print what will most affect you, which, from the informatics point of view, are in sections 1173 and 1174.

Standardization of information systems plays a large role in this legislation to simplify and ensure the portability of health care insurance from one employer and payer to another. Accountability depends on those same data standards to allow comparisons of processes and outcomes of care across health plans, providers, communities, states, and regions. In fact, without standardized data describing patients and their treatments, there can be no comparisons of their outcomes of care or of the processes used to treat them.

With standardization comes the advent of national comparative studies of health care outcomes. The outcomes will be simple and primarily financial, such as charges per visit and charges per stay. But when providers submit most claims electronically with standardized formats, we will begin to study charges per capita per year and charges per person per month, as health plans do now.

While portability of insurance will relieve some of the worries of changing employers, the accountability part of the legislation will help transform medicine and spawn innumerable outcome studies from vast observational databases. True, the data may not be as clinical, detailed, or clean as those collected in funded clinical research trials, but they will cover the practices and financial outcomes of millions of Americans in ordinary medical practice. Patients in funded research trials number in the hundreds or thousands, are carefully screened, and are not in an ordinary medical setting. The observational databases our society will build will include clinical and financial data on millions of Americans.

Let's look at the details of this legislation as it applies to information requirements. Sections 1173 and 1174 include the following language:

SECTION 1173. (a) STANDARDS TO ENABLE ELECTRONIC EXCHANGE—

1. IN GENERAL—The Secretary shall adopt standards for transactions, and data elements for such transactions, to enable health information to be exchanged electronically, that are appropriate for: (A) the financial and administrative transactions described in paragraph (2); and (B) other financial and administrative transactions determined appropriate by the Secretary, consistent with the goals of improving the operation of the health care system and reducing administrative costs.

2. TRANSACTIONS—The transactions referred to in paragraph (1A) are transactions with respect to the following: (A) Health claims or equivalent encounter information. (B) Health claims attachments. (C) Enrollment and disenrollment in a health plan. (D) Eligibility for a health plan. (E) Health care payment and remittance advice. F) Health plan premium payments. (G) First report of injury. (H) Health claim status. (I) Referral certification and authorization.

The legislation proposes to standardize for electronic automation insurance claims for the fee-for-service community; encounter forms from providers who receive capitation; supporting documentation usually attached to claims; enrollment and disenrollment notification between employers and plans; eligibility notification between health plans and providers; health care payment and remittance advice between payers and providers; health plan premium payments between employers and insurers; first report of injury between providers and payers, and perhaps with employers; insurance claim status between payers and inquiring providers or members; and referral certification and authorization between payers and providers.

The legislation purports to automate financial transactions. They are easier to automate than clinical data, because they are far simpler and more standardized. Nevertheless, first report of injury will require coding the injuries and their causes, including clinical details, and referral certification and authorization will include clinical information, as well as diagnosis and procedure codes.

For instance, clinician requests for prior approval by utilization management agencies for many expensive procedures will be followed by a series of computer-prompted questions from precertification clerks about criteria related to expected symptoms and results of diagnostic tests and therapeutic trials. Will the information content of those utilization management algorithms be standardized for national distribution, as is the jargon of most electronic banking transactions?

Portability of information requires moving information electronically in standard format, rather than by paper. For insurance and clinical information to become truly portable, we need the same identifier numbers for patients and providers. Now, every new patient who arrives at a health care provider receives a new medical record number.

How many medical records do you have? By recalling all the health care providers who have treated me, including the hospital in which I was born, where I was treated in emergency departments, or received surgery, plus the physicians who have seen me in their offices, the health clinics at schools where I studied, and the myriad dentists who have cleaned my teeth, I estimate I have about 30 medical records—and 30 medical record numbers. Those medical records exist in states from Washington, DC, to California and from Massachusetts to Florida.

Then I thought of the claims records that I must have in insurers' databases—inpatient claims, outpatient claims, dental claims. There must be more insurance numbers for me than medical record numbers. How would we ever integrate all those data in all those paper records to study the resources used to diagnose and treat my unremarkable collection of minor ailments and preventive health visits over more than 40 years? We could not do so cost-effectively.

How can a nation promote "accountability" in health care practice if it cannot aggregate data about treatments for multiple people at multiple locations over time? With paper records, we could not do so. The two keys to integrating those data for accountability studies involve standardizing the way we identify individuals in providers' medical record and accounting systems and in payers' claims processing systems and then standardizing the data collected at all locations of care, and transmitted between providers and payers.

Section 1173 (a) of the legislation states the goal of standardizing basic transactional data now collected at almost every meeting of a provider with a patient. These data will include some clinical details about injuries and prior approval of some medical services. But how do we identify patients and health plan members if every payer and provider assigns a different record number for each individual? Section 1173 (b) takes care of this problem, at least in theory:

(b) UNIQUE HEALTH IDENTIFIERS:

1. IN GENERAL—The Secretary shall adopt standards providing for a standard unique health identifier for each individual, employer, health plan, and health care provider for use in the health care system. In carrying out the preceding sentence for each health plan and health care provider, the Secretary shall take into account multiple uses for identifiers and multiple locations and specialty classifications for health care providers.

2. USE OF IDENTIFIERS—The standards adopted under paragraph (1) shall specify the purposes for which a unique health identifier may be used.

Congress intends for every American to have a number, presumably from birth, which will be his or her medical record number. When I visit a health care provider in the near future, I will give the physician my medical record number, instead of being issued a new one by the physician's office. Similarly, every payer will use the same number for processing claims for me.

Because I am a physician, I will have a unique provider number, too. I will use it on all claims I generate for my patients. Urgent care centers, nursing homes, hospitals, ambulatory surgery centers, home health agencies, chiropractors, and optometrists will have such numbers as well.

The National Committee on Vital and Health Statistics recommends that a new number, not the social security number, be used for the medical record number for each American, and that a new number, not the Uniform Physician Identification Number (UPIN), be used for physicians.

In the legislation, Congress charges the National Committee on Vital and Health Statistics with the job of advising the Secretary of Health and Human Services about the regulations to implement the legislation. The committee was to have completed its work and recommended specific regulations to the Secretary of HHS no later than 18 months after the passage of the legislation, which was signed in August 1996, so the due date for the regulations was in late February 1998. The regulations have not been implemented in late 1998 because Congress has not passed legislation to determine how to keep electronic medical records private. Who sits on this committee? The legislation states that:

1. The members of the Committee shall be appointed from among persons who have distinguished themselves in the fields of health statistics, electronic interchange of health care information, privacy and security of electronic information, population-based public health, purchasing or financing health care services, integrated computerized health information systems, health services research, consumer interests in health information, health data standards, epidemiology, and the provision of health services. Members of the Committee shall be appointed for terms of 4 years.

Members of the committee come from the community of specialists in health services research and leadership positions in health care organizations. Most have strong academic credentials. Don E. Detmer, MD, was Vice President and Chancellor of the University of Virginia Medical Center in Charlottesville before he took a sabbatical to study health care information systems around the world and security issues for digital information management systems. This prepared him well for his appointment as committee chairman by Secretary Shalala. He holds a part-time faculty appointment at the University of Virginia and an endowed chair at the business school of Cambridge University, England. The committee maintains a Web site where you can find all its deliberations, as well as its subcommittee and brief biographies of the committee members. The URL for the web site is http://aspe.os.dhhs.gov/ncvhs.

Many committee members were involved in the study of the feasibility of computer-based patient records produced by the Institute of Medicine of the National Academy of Sciences at the request of Congress. The study, which was completed in 1991, essentially found that there are no technological impediments today to a national, standardized, computer-based patient record. The only impediments, which are enormous, are economic and political. In other words, we do not know how to mandate the standards for the data or how to pay for the infrastructure, but the technology per se is not the problem. The results of the study were published by the National Academy Press in 1991 in *The Computer-Based Patient Record: An Essential Technology for Health Care*. Not coincidentally, Detmer also served as chairman of that committee. A second edition of the book, updated with chapters about legislative and technical trends promoting computer-based patient records, appeared in early 1998.

What are the implications of this legislation? You can probably imagine a major one already. When patients and health plan members bring their identification numbers with them, the information systems of all providers and insurers will have to accept them. For the health care community, this conversion to a new scheme for identifying patients will be much more challenging than the monumental "year 2000" problem has been to date. The software will need sophisticated logic to make sure others in the system do not have the same ID number. Because these new ID numbers will be the most important data in those information systems, preventing duplicates is paramount.

In the information systems of most large hospitals and health care insurers, there are people with the same social security number and same name. But the information system assigns a unique number to each, so it can control how the numbers are assigned. In fact, the same person may have multiple numbers assigned for multiple separate visits when his or her medical record was not available. But when the patients bring the numbers with them, how does the provider ascertain if the number presented is valid? How does it determine that there are not two patients with the same number in the system, including patients who have not been seen in a number of years and whose data may not be immediately accessible by the core transaction system? These and many other issues will keep the health care and insurance industries busy for a long time.

What about accountability? With the advent of electronic communication of so much standardized data; robust and inexpensive hardware and software technologies to store the data; the advent of World Wide Web standards for distribution, encryption, and easy access (with proper identification) to the data; and standardized identification numbers to make longitudinal and comprehensive databases possible, we will see a flowering of analysis of observational data on a massive national scale.

Profiling outcomes and processes of care will give us a national laboratory for the study of efficacy and efficiency of various health care services and health care providers. We will profile how physicians and allied health professionals practice and how patients consume resources. We will profile both suppliers and demanders of health care services. We will learn an extraordinary amount of valuable information about which processes work, and which do not work, to achieve desired health care outcomes.

But at what price? One articulate objection to the legislation came from Beverly Woodward in an article entitled "Intrusion in the Name of 'Simplification,'" in the *Washington Post*:

"The beneficiaries of this system will in fact be the commercial enterprises that have been promoting it and that will reap large-scale gains from it, principally information technology vendors and health care insurers. For the vendors of information technology, a national health care data system is a bonanza and will bring billions in sales. Insurers stand to gain because they will be able to track patients and use this information to control their risks through such means as the manipulation of policy coverage and stringent utilization management techniques. In the eyes of the industry, information management has become the key to risk management."[1]

Woodward is correct that information management is the key to risk management. She is right, too, that vendors may enjoy a windfall by upgrading their systems for their customers to accommodate these new numbers for patients, members, and providers. Insurers will benefit by finding the cost substantially reduced to link claims from disparate sources, such as hospitals, physicians' offices, and pharmacies into one longitudinal database for retrospective analysis of providers' practice habits and patients' consumption habits. She worries that the leaders of the National Committee on Vital and Health Statistics have much more incentive to design a system that maximizes the availability of observational data for retrospective analysis than one that minimizes the risk of invasion of privacy of citizens.

Congress will determine legislation to protect the privacy of Americans' medical records. The legislation, and regulations derived from it, will tell us how our privacy will fare in the era of electronic medical records and large clinical databases. The legislation is wending its way through Congress. The National Committee on Vital and Health Statistics will not determine privacy protection. Legislation not yet written in late 1998 will do that.

## Reference

1. Woodward, B. "Intrusion in the Name of 'Simplification.'" *Washington Post*, Aug. 15, 1996, p. A19.

# Chapter 16
## Information in a System-Oriented World

A *patient—whether he or she telephones or arrives in person at a walk-in clinic, physician's office, ambulatory diagnostic center, or hospital—can be quickly identified as someone we have serviced before or as a brand-new customer. The patient's laboratory tests and imaging results can be transported electronically as he or she is referred within the system, thus eliminating the need for costly and inconvenient repetition of diagnostic tests.*

*The same information can be viewed simultaneously by members of a quickly formed team of specialists functioning in separate locations but able to consult about the diagnosis and course of treatment for complex cases. Documented quality outcomes demonstrate continuous improvement in all system locations.*

*New economic relationships formed by previously independent system members have eliminated the incentives to provide care in any setting except one that is most appropriate and cost-effective. Perverse incentives under capitation also have been resolved. Employers seek out the system with custom-designed benefit packages that fully satisfy their employees and are also affordable.*

This is the future vision of one of the leading regional health care systems in the nation, with headquarters in New Mexico. The vision was defined by focus groups of its customers—patients, family members, or other individuals interested in the welfare of specific patients—and the employers or governments that pay the health care bills. What emerged from the focus sessions was that customers want more than health. They want to have a say in how the processes of care and mending are organized and financed.

What will it take to make this vision, these customers' goals, a reality? For ambitious health care systems, achieving these goals requires a fundamental shift in management focus and allocation of capital from facilities for treatment of existing diseases to information technologies linking those facilities and all providers.

Integrated regional health care systems of the future will need far fewer expensive pieces of diagnostic equipment and fewer inpatient facilities than have been supported by the current way of financing medical care services. But the investments that regional systems will have to make in information and communication technologies will be larger than the current, fragmented medical marketplace of independent, small medical groups and hospitals has installed to date.

When financing of health care changes from fee for service, paid to independent providers by indemnity insurance, to capitation, paid to integrated regional health care systems by employers and governments, the principal focus of providers will switch from revenue management to cost management. And the most important technological assets of the providers will change from technologies for which they can bill for services to technologies to help them measure and manage their use of resources most effectively.

There will be less emphasis on magnetic resonance scanners, sleep disorder centers, and operating rooms and more attention on transaction, analysis, and communication systems. These information technologies represent the nervous system of the successful regional integrated health care system.

## Connecting Links

What technologies will physicians, managers, and board members of an ambitious, organized care system use to satisfy their customers' wishes, as defined in the scenario above? To quickly identify a person as someone new to the system of care or someone who has been treated at any of the points of care in the system requires:

- A telecommunication network linking all the points of care (for fast electronic communication).
- A database (in which data about all previous patients and customers of the delivery system are stored) readily available from any of those points of care.

Paper records and voice communication cannot offer the efficiency and the convenience of an electronic database of customers' and patients' demographic and clinical information available online to all points of care, with patients' and health plan members' records stored according to a master person index that uniquely identifies every individual. Of course, to access the master person index and database requires that providers who want to share it standardize their personal computer equipment and software to use the system.

When customers are recognized at point of service and their records are obtainable electronically, they do not have to complete lengthy forms at each encounter with their health care system—and providers do not feel compelled to repeat diagnostic tests they might have repeated had paper records of those previous tests not been available.

Beyond the initial contact, the organized health care delivery system needs patient care information systems at all inpatient and outpatient locations of service to collect clinical data in standardized formats, using a standardized nomenclature for diagnoses and procedures. In this way, an electronic medical record can be created over time. That computer-based patient record will be contained in a distributed relational database and maintained by a relational database management system.

This computer-based patient record will be the integrated regional health care system's most valuable asset, because it is the principal resource for facilitating care of individual patients and for informing the continuous quality improvement efforts of the system as a whole. In addition to clinical and demographic data, this computer-based patient record can and should include satisfaction and functional status information to permit outcomes management for factors other than cost, mortality, or untoward comorbidities.

## Three Kinds of Information Technology
Overall, three categories of information technology will be indispensable to successful regional health care systems. The most familiar to everyone are the transaction systems that permit real-time updates of electronic databases for individual customers and patients. Admission, scheduling, order entry, results reporting, and laboratory and radiology systems are all transaction systems.

The second type of information technology is the analytical or decision-support system. These are relatively new to health care organizations because costs of care have not been important until recently. Decision-support systems include cost accounting, market research, executive information, and ad hoc query systems. All depend on large databases of patients' records to permit interrogation of the data to find important trends in outcomes and processes of care that indicate where opportunities may exist to improve service.

The third category of information technology is the communication system—local- and wide-area networks and metropolitan area networks—that permit electronic communication of data about customers and patients among many hundreds or thousands of separate locations of care.

Together, transaction and communication systems permit rapid flow of current information about patients (customers), and analytical and decision support systems facilitate surveillance of the processes and outcomes of care for opportunities for improvement.

## Telemedicine
Communication systems are especially valuable to a distributed organized care system. They permit communication of a patient's computer-based record from one location to another, and they allow multiple locations to access the record simultaneously. They facilitate the flow of data from points of care to databases for analysis and planning.

Communication systems can carry more than textual information. The newer network architectures, with wider bandwidth, permit communication of physicians' dictation, pathology and radiology images, and video images of cardiac catheterizations and of abdominal or pelvic ultrasound studies. They even enable communication of full motion, full color video images from endoscopic surgery, so that an expert in such surgery can watch and consult on a procedure performed by a physician without as much experience, even though the two physicians may be 100 or 1,000 miles apart.

Teleconferencing and telemedicine may begin to reduce the travel and inconvenience that customers of health care services often experience when they must visit several consultants at different locations, carrying their records with them from appointment to appointment.

Needed, too, are the databases and large-capacity optical storage devices to archive all those images in electronic form. Optical storage replaces the film library. Picture archiving and communication systems manage the storage and retrieval of images. High-resolution digital workstations replace view boxes and hot lights.

Telecommunication systems promise for organized care systems some of the conveniences and efficiencies that large multispecialty group practices have always been able to provide their patients—the benefit of having many physicians, of various specialties, practicing in the same setting, and sharing a common scheduling system and a common medical record.

To take advantage of all these new and rapidly improving information technologies, the organized care system needs to do several things:

- Agree to standard policies, procedures, and record-keeping rules.
- Invest in integrated transaction and communication systems.
- Fund the training of all staff to use those information and communication systems appropriate for them.

The investments organized care systems make in information technologies will be the most important investments they will ever make. These information and communication systems will be seen as the systems' principal assets, after the people using them. The leaders of organized care systems must be familiar with these technologies and their uses in order to guide their organizations to prudent decisions about what will be multimillion-dollar strategic investments.

## Organized Care versus Managed Care

The goals of an organized care system can be distinguished easily from those of a managed care system organized by insurers.

In the latter, there is usually little or no coordination of care by the providers themselves, except that accomplished by primary care gatekeepers. The physicians and hospitals involved are kept separate by the insurer. The insurer is the middleman who orchestrates the selection, governance, and rewarding of providers. But insurers generally have not been effective middlemen, because they have remained claims-paying bureaucracies and outsiders who have tended to throw a pall of regulatory micro-management over providers without helping them reorganize to deliver better and more disciplined services.

Insurers usually invest in infrastructure only insofar as is necessary to process claims, contract with individual providers, and market health insurance products that depend on the provider networks they establish. Providers have nothing in common with one another except the insurer with whom they have contracts.

Control of health care costs depends on discounts from providers, perhaps primary care capitation and per diems or case rates with hospitals, and on all the variations of the theme of utilization review. Fundamentally, providers do not manage these delivery systems. The payers do.

In contrast to managed care, which tends to produce hideously inefficient bureaucracies for insurers and frustrating impediments to practice for physicians, "organized care" permits providers to organize and govern themselves, and probably to obtain the insurance functions as well. The regional integrated health care system of the future, one that includes physicians and hospitals as well as other providers and facilities, will be organized into a self-disciplined team for care. It will resemble the delivery systems of the large regional medical group practices, such as Geisinger Clinic and Health Plan in central Pennsylvania.

Organized care depends on group practice and shared capital and governance with hospitals. Providers govern themselves with data. They have the common purpose and capital to invest in information and telecommunication systems to make their systems of care achieve some of the efficiencies of group practices. And they govern their costs by corporate culture and shared values as well as shared information.

Many emerging regional health care systems are now investing in the information technologies that will allow them to satisfy their customers and wrest control of their operations from insurers.

# Section III

## New Structures for Health Care Delivery

# Chapter 17
## The Organized Health Care System

By nature, health care is a regional business. People who live in metropolitan and urban areas of our country usually obtain health care services within their immediate geographic areas.

As a natural response to increasing specialization, expensive technologies, and mounting competition, providers of direct patient care are forming regional health care systems. Physicians, facilities, and other health care services are migrating to organized systems of care that share financial and insurance risks involved in caring for the people within a community.

An organized, regional health care network can include half a dozen hospitals, hundreds of physicians, and a battery of complementary health care services, such as home health care, nursing home services, and urgent care. All these providers unite to accept contracts from large buyers of their services, such as corporations that purchase health care for employees. The organized system assumes the financial risks of delivering comprehensive services to a defined population, under a budget set in direct contract with the community's employers or insurers.

In time, all health care providers may assemble in these regional integrated systems. In fact, the most effective and efficient U.S. health care delivery systems are large, capitated, multispecialty group practices. Of these practices, perhaps the best known are the Permanente Medical Groups of Kaiser Health Plans, which have been practicing organized care for more than 50 years.

Organized care integrates the many providers of health care so they are all accountable for a patient's total care. It inspires health care providers to improve the quality, efficiency, and effectiveness of their services and encourages them to offer comprehensive care at the lowest possible cost.

When physicians and hospitals unite in integrated systems, they can determine which other providers will work with them in their regional network. The system's members share financial risk. Together, they invest in outpatient diagnostic and treatment facilities and information and communication systems that help manage patient populations over time, under a set budget.

In addition to policies and procedures, organized networks are managed by culture. When providers form an organized network, they naturally join others who share their values and approaches to care delivery. Because all members of the system share a standard way of doing business, an organized network reduces the need for systematic and intensive utilization review. Within Kaiser and the military health system, far less utilization management takes place than among providers contracting with managed care insurers.

## System Evolution

Compared with hospitals, nursing homes, home health care agencies, and diagnostic and ambulatory surgery centers, physicians are the least organized. They have great difficulty pooling capital to create the organizational infrastructure of organized care. Therefore, hospitals usually catalyze the grouping of physicians into regional group practices that can in turn cooperate with regional groups of hospitals and other health care facilities. The result: An organized system makes all providers share the economic and management responsibilities involved in caring for a defined population of people over time.

You may think that my concept of provider-sponsored organized care systems is fantasy—wishful thinking at best. You may discount the examples of Group Health of Puget Sound, Henry Ford Health System, Geisinger Health System, and the Mayo Clinic and Health System as anomalies in a much larger world of fragmented, disorganized, intensely independent medical groups. The payers will always have a role in organizing and managing care, because most physicians cannot agree to share capital and management to create organized care systems. You may be right. But I hope that the profession of medicine recognizes its opportunity to lead the management of the health of populations the way in which it leads the treatment of disease in individuals.

No one would deny that professionals of most types are organizing into larger firms—law, accounting, engineering, advertising, investment, consulting. They contract with corporations for work. So, too, are clinicians aggregating into medical firms—MedPartners, PhyCor, Tenet, American Psych Management, multispecialty group practices, IPAs, PHOs, MSOs, and OWAs (other weird arrangements).

So, when will clinical professionals take over the management of health care organizations of professionals? The transition continues. It is happening. Hospitals that acquire single-specialty primary care groups do so to control referrals to subspecialists who admit patients to their inpatient facilities. Hospitals won't build multispecialty groups for fear of alienating subspecialist physicians they might not select for their groups. Hospitals discover that acquired primary care groups do not produce enough revenue to pay for their costs and find they need to subsidize those groups at $20,000-100,000 per doctor per year. Hospitals usually pay too much for those groups and then lose many productive physicians in them to retirement.

The most stable group practices are multispecialty groups in which an income distribution formula redistributes income from procedural physicians to primary care physicians who follow patients over time. The physicians in these groups understand the need for income sharing, because the fee-for-service model of care so disproportionately favors proceduralists financially. Hospitals cannot risk alienating subspecialists, they believe, so they acquire primary care practices that do not produce enough income to support the salaries the hospital agrees to pay the primary care physicians to entice them to sell their practices.

This painful subsidization cannot continue indefinitely. Physicians will organize in medical firms and contract for readily available hospital beds when they need them.

-

# Chapter 18
## Informatics for the Transition from Managed Care to Organized Care

In the transition from managed care to a system of organized care in which providers accept responsibility for both the financing and the delivery of care, a key ingredient will be information systems that speed the flow of accurate and up-to-date records about health plan members. Insurance companies may hold the key to the capital and the standards to create computer-based patient records.

By managed care, I mean health care services sold to employers as health insurance benefits for their employees, characterized by a delivery system of independent providers contracting with a health insurer. Beneficiaries of the health insurance can obtain all the benefits of the health insurance as long they follow the rules of the insurance and see providers approved by the managed care plan. Providers have little, or nothing, in common except for the contracts they have signed to participate in the delivery system of the insurer. The network of providers and the insurance benefits available to beneficiaries are defined by the insurer. The insurer manages the network. Providers and beneficiaries play by the rules dictated to them by the insurer.

The insurer usually charges the employer for utilization management services, including preadmission certification, concurrent review, and retrospective analysis of claims, to "manage" providers and control their tendencies to treat patients with too many services. To my way of thinking, managed care is hideously inefficient from the point of view of the delivery system. Sure, the insurers bargain with providers with covered lives and providers give up discounts off their retail fees to participate in the insurer's network, and some of the savings are passed along to employers. And, yes, utilization management may reduce the number of unnecessary tests and procedures ordered by physicians, but at a large administrative cost to providers that is not passed along to the buyers of services. Is there a better way to organize health care services?

I call the better way organized care, as opposed to managed care. In organized care, the middleman role that the insurer plays, the role of organizing providers, supervising their services, and managing services for members, is disintermediated, and providers organize and govern themselves, with information and shared values, to satisfy the requirements of the buyers of health insurance—the employer and its employees. The insurer adds value as long as no other entity can organize a network of providers; print membership materials; staff a telephone pool to answer questions of beneficiaries, patients, and providers; process claims; and arrange financing when the employer is not self-insured. These administrative functions can be performed by a provider organization, obviating the need for the insurer in the equation at all. When I say organized care system (OCS), I mean an organization of providers that has acquired the administrative wherewithal to manage the clinical and financial responsibilities of a health care insurer and to contract directly with employers in its location. Witness the marketplace for health care in the Twin Cities of Minnesota. Organized delivery systems of providers have driven third-party health care insurers from the market.

There will be a role for the large health insurers with national scope for many years to come, because large employers want to deal with one insurer, not a multitude of separate organized care systems in various parts of the country. But for most Americans, employed by firms with one location of operation, the local organized care system will become more and more appealing. Getting the insurer out of the middle of the health care transaction between buyers of health insurance, beneficiaries of that insurance, and providers will eliminate considerable cost in inefficient communication and the bureaucracy built up by the middleman function.

For providers to perform effectively and efficiently, without the insurer in the way, they need to know one another and share an efficient means of communicating with one another about patients, about the insurance program purchased by the employer, and about the past ailments of patients and the services rendered to them by the delivery system. What sort of information processing do providers need in order to take on the insurers' administrative and financial roles? In addition to the insurers' traditional roles, what information do providers need to manage their patients well and to support preventive health activities for their members and continuous quality improvement activities for themselves? What information do providers need to care for patients better than they have in the past?

Providers are moving from producing procedures at single points in time and being managed in a minimal way by annoying external insurance companies to managing the care of populations of people over time and managing themselves in a thorough and comprehensive way to maximize the quality of health care services they produce for their members. Providers are working together, depending on each other to produce good outcomes, and not as isolated as they were in managed care, when the insurance company was the intermediary. In order to carry the level of performance to the next higher plane, above the realm of managed care, providers need to act and work in concert. They need to incorporate the concept of primary care provider, not as a gatekeeper but as a conductor or orchestrator of the services made available to patients. They need to share information about their patients quickly to expedite and improve care and to produce the opportunity for systematic study of the results of their work to allow them to improve quality over time.

The OCS needs claims processing; coordination of benefits; enrollment and membership services; ways of keeping accurate records of the providers who are a part of the network; credentialing records; practice guidelines that have been adopted by the organization; rules for certification of certain procedures; and rules for case management, utilization review, and

## Informatics for the Transition from Managed Care to Organized Care

home health care treatment. The OCS needs the same kinds of information services that a managed care system needs, but providers will be using their information systems to help them manage their own services rather than having their services policed by an outside entity that does not put information at their fingertips. The OCS needs practice management capabilities for scheduling patients for care and recording the serviced rendered to them; risk management systems to control the financial risk that goes with the role of OCS; and data on all the services rendered to patients and all the clinical findings from physicians' examinations and laboratory studies for on-line, real-time patient care and for retrospective clinical and health services research analysis.

Providers put all this information at their fingertips with standardized and shared office practice systems; computer-based patient records; and insurance-oriented managed care information systems that are impossible to implement in a setting in which providers are independent of one another, do not share governance or financial risk for the care of defined populations of patients, and are "coordinated" by multiple third-party insurers.

In order to share a computer-based patient record, providers must agree to standardize the data definitions they use and their means of collecting data about their members and their patients. Standardizing on vendors' software and hardware makes the work of integrating data simpler, but the key to successful sharing of data is standardizing data definitions. Providers in an OCS want to share information about health plan members and patients easily. To do so, the technological barriers to data transfer among incompatible systems must be eliminated (by very hard work and considerable capital). Without a shared organizational structure that allows participating providers to pool and share capital for information systems, to establish standards and mandate adherence to them, and to share a staff of information systems experts to implement them, it will be impossible to share computer-based patient records.

The principal competitive advantages that providers in an OCS have that will help them compete successfully with managed care systems controlled by insurers are computer-based patient records. Insurer-dominated delivery systems cannot implement CPRs without employing providers and funding the information infrastructure. Will providers have the capital, and the political wherewithal to use it, to develop their own shared information infrastructure for computer-based patient records? Frankly, probably not, except in the case of the largest group practices. The cohesive culture and extraordinary leadership needed to establish information standards that all providers will share do not exist yet in most health care organizations. But there is another alternative, and it may define the future role of insurers in organized care.

The alternative is for an insurer to merge with a selected delivery system of providers. Over time, the providers will begin to behave like an organized care system, with the insurer as a partner rather than an overseer. The insurer begins to act less like an outside entity harassing providers and more like a systems integrator, bringing the capital and expertise to provide the information systems for the delivery network.

The Kaiser Permanente health care organization, an organized care system that is more than 60 years old, includes physicians in the Permanente Medical Group; a health plan in the Kaiser Health Plan; and, in California, an extensive network of health care treatment facilities, including hospitals, managed by the Hospitals Division. This organization is planning to spend several billion dollars on information systems to give physicians in all its service locations access to computer-based patient records. With this infrastructure, the organization can move information about patients to clinicians more quickly and more accurately than by paper, can increase the velocity and consistency of care throughout the system, and can promulgate practice guidelines that the physicians themselves have adopted. This system will not be imposed on providers by an outside policing entity. The electronic system of patient information, and automated advice to clinicians, will be designed by and for clinicians to help them work more efficiently and effectively.

Most providers are not organized into entities they control. They are organized into delivery systems by payers. Over time, to reduce their operating costs, payers will reduce the number of physicians with whom they contract and will work cooperatively with those who treat patients best and have the best outcomes of care. To cut their own costs of doing business, physicians will prefer to work with fewer managed care plans, the ones that give them the most patients and that treat them best. Therein lie the seeds of a symbiotic relationship. Traditional indemnity insurers don't want to go out of business and see their customers move to organized care systems such as Kaiser. Physicians do not want to see all their patients migrate in the same direction. So, to compete, physicians and insurers will collaborate, until their working relationship resembles that of Kaiser. As the Permanente Medical Group grows, physicians in it feel less like partners and more like employees. So, too, with physicians affiliated with Blue Cross, or Aetna, or MetroHealth. Eventually, most physicians will ally with one delivery network or another, just as retailers have learned the value of franchises and market standards.

So we have come full circle. We started with insurers creating managed care plans, keeping physicians independent of each other and practicing in delivery networks in which physicians are "managed" by utilization review and the requirement for prior approval of expensive services. Now we are moving to a time when physicians almost "marry" one insurer or another to gain access to computer-based patient records that in most communities only insurers have the wherewithal to define and capitalize. The entire premise that providers and insurers will find the reason to marry their efforts depends on the importance of capital and standards in the establishment of computer-based patient records.

# Chapter 19

# Key Success Factors for Organized Care Systems

In this chapter, five factors that will be critical to the success of organized care systems are described. These factors are of universal concern to integrated health care systems, especially those being formed from regional systems of not-for-profit hospitals.

If organized care systems (OCSs) are to replace managed care organizations as we know them, or at least compete successfully with already existing and well-financed health care delivery systems, they will have to attract physicians, reduce costs, develop effective governance structures, implement financial and information systems aimed at computerized medical records, and overcome the hospital culture from which they have sprung.

■ **Attract and retain primary care physicians and selected subspecialists to fill voids in specific geographic regions covered by the OCS.**

The OCS needs to attract physicians to join its delivery system and to stay in the system once they have joined. The OCS needs to identify all the benefits to physicians of locating in communities it serves and to demonstrate what it can do to reduce the costs physicians incur in relocating to those communities and operating practices there. The OCS needs to understand that physicians become most loyal to the sources of their patients, whether they come from within a group practice, from other satisfied patients, from independent physicians outside the practice, from managed care firms with whom they have contracts, or from employers under contract. Hospitals and hospital systems usually cannot deliver patients, especially to primary care physicians with outpatient practices. On the other hand, the OCS can channel members of its health plan to physicians. The OCS does have a means, probably more than one, to direct patients to selected physicians. Physicians, like the rest of us, consider whether to move to a community, or whether to remain in a community, on the basis of job satisfaction and security, their sense of value in that community, their influence in contracting decisions that will effect their future income, and the support system offered to them and their families. Traditionally, the most successful group practices have been adept at recruiting and retaining physicians. The OCS needs to learn, and take guidance, from its successful group practices and defer to them in the recruitment of physicians.

## ■ Reduce the costs of delivering excellent care within the OCS.

Increasing proportions of the OCS's total revenue will come from capitated contracts, in which revenue is fixed and costs must be managed well, and less from discounted fee for service. The OCS is not homogeneous. Within the OCS, hospitals are still paid discounted fee for service for the large majority of patients, while medical groups may receive more than half their revenue through capitated contracts. A conflict of incentives between hospitals and medical groups must be overcome. The OCS needs to take the longer view that capitation as a form of payment will increase in importance and prevalence for the foreseeable future. In spite of political inclinations to the contrary, the OCS needs to act like a constellation of group practices. It also needs to give information to physicians as promptly, accurately, and completely as possible, showing them how their practice habits and patients' outcomes compare to those of their peers. With these data, the OCS can begin to function as a learning organization for its clinicians, allowing them to learn from each other and to improve their work together. This is not a familiar habit to most hospitals. If they are involved in total quality improvement, it is usually for service quality improvement. Countless committee meetings are spent reducing the time tissue samples take to reach laboratories, increasing the palatability of food for patients, reducing retakes of x-ray studies, or increasing the speed with which interoffice mail moves through the system.

Each of those projects may have merit, and they may all make participating administrators proud. However, the 80:20 rule screams out the need for better data about processes of care and outcomes for patients in the hands of clinicians and for an organizational structure that rewards time spent by clinicians in redesigning processes of care. The time and resources consumed in service quality improvement studies, including the training of managers for them, must be matched, at least, by investment in information systems, health services and clinical research technologies, and staff to analyze data and by incentives for clinicians to participate in continuing clinical quality improvement studies. That's where the money is, not in making the mail move faster, the meals taste better, or tissue samples reach the laboratory sooner.

## ■ Develop a governance structure to promote the success of the OCS.

The OCS needs a governance structure to free it from the tyranny of disaffected minorities when the majority wants to accomplish something the minority opposes. A federal form of governance may be suitable, and necessary. In federalism, suggestions about management of the organization may well percolate up from the operating units. Agreement on standards for clinical practice, managed care contracting, financial accounting, and information systems implementation may be developed, should be developed, in the operating units. Once the most influential governing body of the organization votes to adopt those standards, the separate operating units, including group practices, must adhere to them. If this discipline is not in place, there can be no hope of creating an integrated health care system or the integrated information infrastructure on which the integrated health care system depends. Computer systems of any kind need precise data definitions and specific data collected in specific ways, meaning the same thing in every location of care.

Think of the chaos that will prevail in managed care contracting if every operating unit is permitted to cut its own deals with purchasers of health care services, insurers, and self-funded employers. The OCS will have no leverage in the marketplace and no means of standardizing its contracts to take advantage of potential economies of scale.

■ **Develop and implement financial and clinical information systems that integrate all components of the OCS electronically to create computer-based patient records.**

The OCS may be one of the largest and most respected integrated health care delivery systems in its region, but it probably faces the daunting task of integrating many disparate transaction and telecommunication systems to create useful electronic data interchange about patients and services rendered to patients. The OCS probably has grown dramatically in hospital facilities and group practices in the past decade but has treated them as parts of a consortium, allowing them to maintain their own transaction systems and databases. Where a number of operating units use the same software vendor for the same functions, they probably have created separate databases at each location, making integration of data across facilities difficult.

The OCS needs to establish a federal form of governance to establish and enforce standards for data definitions, data processing, and data communication among its operating units. Then it needs to define its functional requirements for clinical and financial transaction systems and determine where functional requirements deemed necessary are not now being met. It should concentrate on making those functions available. Assuming that the information systems plan will have as its core goal the creation of a computer-based patient record at every location of care for all patients of the OCS, the implementation plan will include establishing a governance structure for planning and procurement of systems, for budgeting and raising capital, and for selecting and standardizing communication networks and transaction systems. No activity of senior executives, physician leaders, and members of the board is more important than setting up the process for systems planning and procurement to create integrated computer-based patient records for all facilities.

■ **Overcome the culture of hospitals, and create a culture for organized care.**

A culture for organized care must grow. This is a culture that is not of hospitals alone or of physicians and group practices alone. It is of both and also of ancillary health care providers and facilities, melded together to care for populations of people over time, under fixed budgets, at a profit. The only persons licensed to write orders for most medical treatments are physicians, and the operating costs of these organized care systems will be determined largely by their costs. The effectiveness with which physicians manage the myriad therapeutic choices facing them for their patients will make or break the OCS. Medicine is so discretionary that physicians must be leaders of these organized care systems and be held responsible and accountable for their leadership.

With this responsibility must come authority, and therein lies a huge rub, a source of friction among physicians and managers in the OCS. The managers of hospitals control most of the capital assets of the OCS, but physicians control most of the intellectual assets needed to direct the care of patients in the OCS and thereby control the operating costs of the OCS. The culture that emerges cannot maintain this "we" versus "they" mentality—with managers scoffing at physicians for not understanding business and physicians dismissing managers for not understanding medicine. The OCS needs physician managers with authority over the major operating budgets to break that deadly cycle and to produce successful integration of physicians' work into the fabric of the OCS. To succeed in this, the OCS needs to identify physicians who have cast their lot with it and who have merged their assets with it and treat them better than physicians who only contract with it or with its health insurance products. Physicians in an IPA are not equal to physicians who are employees of the OCS.

The OCS needs a mechanism to make operating units financially whole when they are asked to invest their scarce resources for the sake of the larger organization. Without the OCS's funding standardization of information systems, for instance, operating units will be reluctant to invest in standardized systems when existing systems work well for them.

The OCS needs a specific, well-defined, detailed strategic plan so that all leaders—clinicians and others—will know by reading it whether a potential hospital, group practice, HMO, or other business venture should be added to the organization if the opportunity to do so presents itself. Most OCSs have grown by opportunity, not strategy. Defining strategy in detail risks offending constituencies that orbit around not-for-profit hospitals. Without that specificity, however, the organization will squander its capital and good will on unwise acquisitions and have insufficient capital for investment in infrastructure. A big, confused, inefficient OCS is no more sustainable or viable than a small, confused, inefficient OCS. Leaders must remove the confusion with a specific, attainable strategic plan. They must reduce inefficiencies with substantial investment in standardized information systems and clinical process improvement.

Ultimately, the success of the OCS depends on successful, efficient, effective clinical work. Clinicians' need incentives aligned with the rest of the OCS. Clinicians need to lead the OCS. Paying lip service to clinicians and managing in spite of them no longer works. The culture will change from a hotel and insurance business trying to micromanage clinicians from the outside to a clinical business with clinicians inside it responsible and accountable for operating profits or losses of the business.

The OCS needs to attract physicians, and their capital—physicians who will commit their future income and professional satisfaction to the success of the organization. The OCS needs to ask physicians, especially primary care physicians in the same region, what is and is not appealing about joining it. The OCS needs to know what changes it can make to its culture and organization to make joining it more appealing to physicians.

Asking questions like this openly and eagerly will go a long way to signal to those inside and outside the organization that the OCS is serious about becoming a physician-friendly place. Without physicians as allies, sharing common incentives, the OCS is carrion. More entrepreneurial organizations will feed on its carcass until it ceases to exist.

# Chapter 20
## Managed Care Administration

When physicians, hospitals, and allied health professionals bill for services they render, their information processing requirements are relatively simple, at least compared to those who also accept financial risk for the care of some or all of their patients. When payers (insurers or employers) accept financial risk for the health care services of beneficiaries, they usually invest in claims processing; membership tracking; and, under managed care, utilization review and provider profiling systems. But payers do not invest in electronic collection of clinical information about beneficiaries, nor do they keep all claims they have processed in electronic form for study after accounts are settled and payments disbursed. In this chapter, we will explore why informatics is so important to capitated organizations and why payers that have traditionally taken financial risk for insuring the health care costs of populations are also learning about informatics.

Capitation requires that providers attend to the health of the populations they serve, in addition to the individuals they treat. They need to process information about the populations for whom they receive capitated payments, information management usually associated with the work of HMOs and insurers: member services, provider credentialing, contracting and profiling, claims adjudication and processing, utilization review, case management, referral tracking, precertification of services, premium billing, funds management, tracking of incurred but not reported claims, marketing, and financial reporting. Employers are also demanding that health plans collect and report data about their operations according to the HEDIS (Health Plan Employer Data and Information set—www.ncqa.org) guidelines. In turn, providers who receive capitation from health plans are expected to collect data on their capitated populations to help the health plans complete the HEDIS reports. A small, but growing number of states mandate that all licensed HMOs report their outcomes according to the HEDIS methodology.

### Member Services
Timely and accurate information on the identity of health plan members is important for both payers and providers. Because members may come and go from the health plan, providers need to know day by day who is eligible for care and who is not. In the past, providers telephoned health plan membership to confirm the eligibility and benefits of every member of a capitated group that they were asked to treat, consuming considerable

resources. Now, happily, wide-area communication networks allow health plans to download changes in their membership rolls to databases accessible by providers with personal computers and modems to allow them to check the eligibility and benefits of members automatically. Health plans must maintain the databases in accurate and current form, or they risk alienating providers. Providers usually cannot obtain payment for services rendered to former health plan members who were not eligible for benefits at the time of care.

A health plan's Member Services department helps members with any difficulties they may have with the health plan or its providers. It is necessary to help members use the plan well, because the plan restricts their access to physicians and other health care services and requires authorization of services. Both restriction of providers and authorization systems take time to learn and skill to use well.

Member Services is responsible for systematically collecting data on member satisfaction and on the incidence and prevalence of medical and administrative problems for members. Structured and standardized surveys are the principal means available to measure the satisfaction of members and to estimate how many have had problems. Automation of Member Services tracking systems aids in retrospective analysis of trends in member satisfaction and helps Member Services complete timely evaluation and resolution of every recorded problem. Automation of complaints from members, including an automatic alerting system for actions that are due (or overdue) by Member Services, reduces the likelihood that members' complaints or problems will "drop between the cracks."

Kongstvedt lists a number of categories for a member contact tracking system*:

- Enrollment issues (selecting or changing PCPs, lost or stolen ID cards, changes in enrollment status).
- Benefit issues (questions about the services of physicians, hospitals, emergency departments, and home health agencies and complaints about levels of benefits).
- Claims issues (in-network and out-of-network claims, denial of claims).
- Plan policies and procedures (primarily about the authorization system).
- Plan administration (rude or unhelpful employees of the health plan).
- Access to care (inability to get an appointment in an appropriate length of time, distance to providers).
- Physician issues (unpleasantness or unhelpfulness).
- Perceived appropriateness and quality of care (inappropriate denial of care, lack of follow-up, delays in diagnosis and treatment).
- Medical office facility issues (unpleasant, dirty, unsafe, or poorly equipped offices).
- Institutional case issues (poorly equipped, unpleasant, unsafe facilities).

---

* Kongstvedt, P. *The Managed Health Care Handbook*, 3rd Edition. Gaithersburg, Md.: Aspen Publishers, 1996, p. 489.

Of utmost importance is an automated information system for logging all contacts with members, including software that helps Member Services complete structured interviews with members to determine the nature of their complaints and what to do about them.

## Financial Accounting and Capitation

Withholds are used in at least 60 percent of HMOs, usually for primary care physicians, to pay for overruns in costs in specialists' and hospitals' charges to the health plan. Physicians need to be aggregated into large risk pools of 50 to 100 physicians, covering thousands of patients, if they are to avoid financial ruin under global capitation from the random distribution of patients with very expensive ailments. For primary care capitation, the financial risks are not so great, and the risk pools do not need to be as large. Nevertheless, capitation withholds and risk pools all require much more sophisticated accounting than is needed by indemnity insurance to pay for fee-for-service medicine. Providers who receive capitation and then subcontract some of the risk to other clinical specialists must be able to account for the flow of funds from the health plan to themselves and to the various clinical groups accepting subcapitation. Accounting must track payments as they are under capitation and as they might have been under fee-for-service, because most clinicians involved in capitation still account for care on a fee-for-service basis and want to know what they would have made under the "normal" payment structure.

The health plan that capitates physicians and group practices needs to maintain stop-loss insurance and have in its contract with physicians specific details of the level of cost for any individual patient and of the aggregate cost of all patients over which additional costs will not be charged against the risk pool. The aggregate level may rise as a physician takes more patients under capitation.

In a similar way, physicians sharing a risk pool for primary care capitation need incentives to minimize the costs of care. In addition to keeping excess funds from primary care capitation, they should share some of the excess funds in the risk pools. To distribute funds to physicians accurately, accounting functions in health plan information systems need to be much more sophisticated than those for fee-for-service payments.

Physicians paid by capitation often wonder how they can make any money seeing sick patients, not recognizing that the capitation payments include funds for members of the health plan assigned to them whom they do not see frequently, if at all. Health plans need to keep encounter records (claims data) from all physicians to show them which members they have treated as patients and the members for which they received capitation payments but did not treat.

Patients fear that they will receive short shrift from physicians with incentives to withhold treatment to save money. Health plans must survey members for their satisfaction with the physicians who treated them to identify cases of medical neglect or negligent treatment. Health plans can predict the numbers of office visits, consultations, hospitalizations, immunizations, and other services by a primary care physician and use their databases of claims to ascertain which physicians are ordering fewer services than expected.

## Administration of Claims and Benefits

Claims processing is the heart and soul of a health plan and a central business activity of any provider organization that tries to manage capitation. Capitated provider organizations that do not process claims are utterly dependent on insurers for information on their encounters with health plan members. Usually, capitated provider organizations acquire information systems to preprocess claims before sending them to the insurer for final adjudication and payment. By preprocessing, they create a database of claims for retrospective study. The organization that owns the claims data has an enormous advantage. Providers who assemble and organize resources for claims preprocessing are much closer to the goal of becoming independent of insurance entities and striking out on their own to contract directly with employers than those that remain dependent on payers for all claims processing.

Claims processing is not simple or inexpensive. It is capital intensive, with robust claims systems (necessary for the variety of contracting terms now in vogue with point-of-service plans) costing $500,000 to $1 million or more for hardware and software, and staff intensive, with a claims adjudicators needed for every 5,000 to 8,000 health plan members. Nevertheless, direct contracting requires providers to manage the claims processing task. Electronic processing of claims and electronic access to claims data by other departments of the health plan, including member services, provider services, and utilization management, are essential to manage health plans efficiently.

Another principal activity of claims processing is to identify other insurers that are liable for some, or all, of individual claims. Effective coordination of benefits can save health plans as much as $5-6 per member per month. Insurers, or third-party administrators, processing claims for beneficiaries of indemnity insurance usually require that information about other insurance coverage be completed on the claim forms.

Many health plans do not require that members submit claims. In fact, it is a marketing advantage that some health plans tout to potential members that they will not have to complete claims. In that case, the providers submit claims but usually do not have information about other insurance coverage. Health plans that do not require members to submit claims must be creative and aggressive in soliciting from members information about their other sources of insurance. Claims departments must also deal with such issues as workers' compensation and subrogation in cases of injury to members by third parties, where other sources of income can offset some, or all, of the costs the health plan would otherwise bear.

Fraud and abuse are frequent bedfellows of claims processing activities. Because so much money flows through claims departments, a small percentage of fraudulent claims may amount to a considerable sum of money. Claims processing operations must be particularly vigilant about controlling who may authorize services, who may create records of providers to whom payments will be made, and who produces and signs checks to providers.

## Medical Records

Under fee-for-service payment arrangements, providers need to schedule patients; keep records of their clinical findings and of the services they render; and send bills, in the form of claims, to patients and/or their payers. While all of these activities can be performed manually, most organizations larger than a single physician's practice use computers and software to maintain financial records. Larger organizations may also use computers for scheduling patients, paying employees and suppliers, and maintaining financial statements. The larger the provider organization, the more likely the presence of automated scheduling and financial systems for preparing bills for services and calculating funds flows, including payroll and bookkeeping. But few, if any, provider organizations keep a database of the claims they have submitted to patients and payers for payment. Few providers keep more than a minimal set of clinical records about their patients in electronic form.

Under fee-for-service arrangements, once a clinical transaction occurs and financial accounts for it are settled, neither provider nor payer has a financial incentive to incur the costs of maintaining electronic records of the transaction. They print their records to paper and free the computer space for current accounting. Every provider organization counts its medical records among its most important possessions. But almost all of those records are on paper, where they may be adequate for retrieving information on individual patients but are totally inadequate for timely health services research studies of the quality and costs of care rendered to populations of patients over time. I predict major investments by both payers and providers in electronic collection of summary claims and clinical data to use in quality improvement and cost reduction studies. Large insurers that are acquiring medical groups all are investing heavily in automated medical record systems.

**Authorization Systems**

Authorization requirements usually affect primary care physicians who want to admit patients to hospitals or send patients to other physicians for consultation. The authorization process is used to review clinical plans for medical necessity, according to guidelines accepted by the plan; to channel care to the most appropriate locations, which often means outpatient treatment for services previously performed in hospitals; to provide timely alerts that patients are approved and scheduled for services that will require concurrent review; and to help the financial department of the health plan anticipate incurred but not reported claims. In tightly controlled health plans, all services not performed by primary care physicians require authorization for payment. In PPOs, where control is not so strict and providers are paid on a fee-for-service basis, authorization requirements may be limited to prior approval for elective hospitalizations, elective surgical procedures, and major diagnostic studies.

For providers to understand that the health plan is serious about maintaining the discipline of prior approval, they must know that their claims for payment, or their capitation payments, without adequate prior approval will be flagged and reduced by some specific amount. The claims processing system must be able to identify services for which prior approval is required, and whether or not prior approval was obtained. Cross-referencing of claims data with utilization management data must be electronic and automatic. The more capable the automated information system is of dealing electronically with unusual circumstances, the faster the processing of financial transactions with providers and the lower the cost of manual claims adjudication. Ideally, the health plan would have an information system for claims and capitation payment so sophisticated that all transactions could be adjudicated automatically and not pended for human inspection and adjudication. There is no such ideal system on the market.

Health plans need authorization systems that allow them to define types of authorization, including prospective authorizations for elective procedures; concurrent authorizations, usually in the case of urgent treatment, such as same-day elective admission to the hospital; and retrospective authorization. Health plans with large numbers of claims pended for review, denied payment because of lack of prior authorization, or given authorization retrospectively have inadequate utilization management programs. Many times, emergency situations warrant treatment before authorization, but large numbers of such services indicate that the authorization process is too cumbersome, too unfamiliar, or too often ignored by providers and/or members. Because timing is important in obtaining authorization, the system must have adequate numbers of telephone lines, adequate numbers of nurses staffing computers and telephones, and adequate training of members and participating physicians about the situations in which to use the authorization system and about the mechanics of using it.

Authorization systems can be based on paper authorization forms, on telephone contact, or on electronic communication between providers and the health plan, with providers entering data directly into the authorization system from personal computers. Paper-based systems only work when the authorization system is controlled by primary care physicians who mail forms to the health plan to inform the claims processing department which claims should be paid in full. When patients choose to make their own referrals and do not engage primary care physicians in those decisions, their claims should be paid at less than the full amount. Keeping track of which claims are approved by PCPs retrospectively may give a health plan insight into which PCPs are active with their patients or not available to their patients.

Telephone-based authorization systems can be a terrible bottleneck and frustration for both members and providers if there are not enough telephone lines and nurses to handle incoming calls. One advantage of telephone authorization systems is that data are collected correctly and more promptly than in paper-based systems. The disadvantage is the frustration providers and members feel in getting approval for services that are almost always approved once they are explained. Nurses staffing a utilization review center need a fast, easy-to-use information system that allows them to navigate through benefits and membership files and retrieve the criteria for approval of any procedure in seconds, so conversation with callers is not interrupted waiting for data to show up on their computer screens.

Authorization systems implemented electronically are more costly, in terms of computer equipment and software at the health plan and at providers' offices. Unlike paper systems, however, electronic systems can track every message reliably, with an audit trail indicating when a message was composed and sent and when and where received. Electronic messages do not get lost in the mail. It is feasible for an electronic system to interact with the provider, suggesting additional data be collected or questions answered. The rule-based logic of an automated authorization system is complex, but it is fairly well-defined for most common elective procedures.

The data elements that any authorization system needs to collect include the member's name, birth date, plan ID number, eligibility status, and primary physician; the referral provider; the date of referral service; diagnoses involved in the treatment decision (in standard ICD-9CM codes); the number of visits to a subspecialist that are approved; and the anticipated discharge date. Nurses using algorithms to estimate the appropriateness of a procedure for which authorization is requested may ask providers more detailed questions about clinical findings or treatment plans.

The health plan must keep accurate records of the locations and qualifications of providers and the terms of the contracts they have signed with the health plan. Payers want a broad

# Managed Care Administration 133

distribution of well-qualified physicians and accredited hospitals available to their beneficiaries. They want to know what proportion of physicians are board-certified and how many physicians work in each zip code in which beneficiaries work and live. They want to know the average driving time between beneficiaries and providers. They want to know that providers will accept payment from the health plan as payment in full. They want to know what proportion of physicians, by specialty, have closed their practices to new patients. The answers to these questions challenge designers of information systems for health plans. The characteristics of participating physicians and facilities, like those of plan members, change too often for publication of accurate paper records. Instead, health plans are beginning to compete for business with employers and providers by offering electronic communication between them.

## Performance Statistics on Physicians

Unfortunately, more health plans treat physicians as adversaries than as partners, and most do not share plan member data in a way that will help physicians change their practice styles. For example, health plans can share members' responses on satisfaction surveys with physicians. They can survey members using health risk assessments and help physicians anticipate risk factors for chronic disease in members assigned to them. Health plans can profile physicians' use of common medical treatments for common ailments and teach them ways of using resources more economically for better patient outcomes. Most health plans send scant comparative reports to physicians, and few, if any, offer analytical staff to ferret out of those data the trends of interest to physicians. I believe that health plans will make those investments as they begin to narrow their provider panels and cultivate partnerships with selected providers, abandoning the adversarial relationship. The relationship between a health plan and its selected providers will become both symbiotic and educational, with the health plan holding most of the data about the processes of care in the community and about the outcomes of care for health plan members and learning to share those data with contracting providers in order to make them more successful.

## Accreditation Activities and Reporting

Employers increasingly want evidence of accreditation before they will consider offering a health plan to employees. A growing minority of states require health plans to pass regular accreditation or face the prospect of losing their licenses. The data collection and reporting requirements of health plans are probably foreign to most physicians and hospital administrators, but they will become important to those who operate health plans.

Health plans face complex and challenging information processing requirements. They are responsible for the total costs of care for populations of people over time and must prove their value to purchasers and regulators not only with competitive prices but also with detailed measures of processes and outcomes that their information systems (manual or automatic) must help them produce. Health plans will succeed if they can garner loyalty and commitment to excellent practice habits of participating providers. Health plans will be more likely to accomplish that goal if they freely and openly share comparative satisfaction, outcomes, and financial data about members with contracting providers, showing them, especially physicians, how they compare to their peers in key measures of clinical quality, productivity, and member satisfaction. The more a health plan uses data to help participating providers perform better, the stronger the health plan will grow in the long run.

# Chapter 21

## Managed Care Information Needs: A Summary Perspective

The key to survival in managed care is management of financial risk. You need to know what is in your contract and what you are obligated to do for which population during which period of time. Information systems can be an enormous help in managing managed care contracts and the financial risks they entail. Poorly selected and configured information systems will do little good for the organization that licenses them. The most important activity of an executive who is moving his or her provider organization into managed care contracting is to lead the process to define the functional requirements for information the organization will need to manage managed care contracts successfully.

Managed care information systems come in many varieties, because managed care is not defined in the same way by any two observers, let alone by any two organizations or software vendors. If your organization is an insurer contracting with one or more IPAs for the medical care of a large population in a given geographic area and you have taken the financial risk for their care under contract with their employers, your information and information technology needs are different from those of a primary care group practice accepting primary care capitation, or of a multispecialty group practice that accepts global capitation and subcontracts part of the capitation to hospitals or specialty groups. A health care organization can manage patients quite well and still suffer financially if it contracts poorly.

What are some of the most important functional requirements for information systems for organizations involved in managed care? Let's consider the needs of group practices, although what follows applies to IPAs and PHOs as well. A group practice usually contracts with an insurer to participate as a provider in a managed care product marketed by the insurer. The group is usually paid discounted fees for services and agrees to accept payment in full from the insurer, without balance billing patients. In this case, the group needs to identify which patients are eligible for the managed care product and determine the utilization management requirements of the product, dealing with preadmission certification, referral notification (or certification), procedures that must be performed on outpatients, and the network of other physicians available for consultation. The group needs to know whom to contact on issues of utilization management and where to send claims in what format. Nowadays, groups must send claims electronically to some insurers just to earn the privilege of contracting with them. The group needs to be able to produce claims for services rendered to patients and include on those claims all information for standard HCFA 1500 claim forms. The group needs standard financial management systems that track remittances and unpaid claims.

Group practices take on additional information processing requirements when they accept payment by capitation. If the payment is for primary care capitation, the group needs to identify eligibility and benefits of patients and account for all services rendered to patients under the contract. Insurers still want capitated providers to submit claims for services. Both insurers and capitated providers need to keep careful records of all the services rendered to capitated patients to estimate whether the capitation has helped or hurt them financially compared to what they would have received from the same insurer, or paid to the same group practice, under discounted fee-for-service arrangements.

If the group practice receives full capitation from an insurer, it still needs to perform many of the information management tasks of an insurer to keep track of all the services rendered to patients, including estimation of incurred but not reported (IBNR) claims. IBNR claims usually are predicted on the basis of consultations and admissions approved by utilization management that have not yet led to claims submitted for payment.

Does the information system of the provider organization support an electronic database of the health benefits of plans with which the group has managed care contracts? Does the system allow providers to check the status of enrollment and eligibility for benefits on-line, without having to place a telephone call to the insurer that invariably is not answered or that is poorly handled by clerks? Does the system have features to support member services, including uniquely identifying each subscriber and member and scheduling coverage termination of members when they reach a certain age or graduate from school? Does the system allow simple and automatic assignment of members to primary care physicians and make it easy to update primary care physician patient rosters when primary care physicians leave, or join, the health plan? Can the system link members with their past health care services, even when they change employers and health plans?

There are many other features of managed care systems to consider. Provider management and services have to do with keeping a current database on physicians, psychologists, physical therapists, radiation oncologists, pharmacies, home health care agencies, and other providers who may participate in a network approved by a health plan. There are as many networks as there are health plans. Even a group practice accepting capitation cannot include within its four walls all the providers needed to care for a population of 10,000 people, and so it must identify extramural providers who contract with it to care for its assigned members. Keeping current records on those providers, and the services they have rendered to the populations served by the group, requires a modern and flexible information system, which, until recently, insurers may have acquired but group practices did not consider.

A capitated group practice also needs to manage utilization. A set of functions for utilization management will be needed, including rules and guidelines that govern intramural and extramural providers. Does the group practice contract with a separate UR firm or manage UR internally? What information systems does the UR firm need? It needs criteria by which review nurses approve or deny permission for services the group has determined need prior approval. It needs databases of participating providers and members. It needs access to claims by members and by providers to verify past services rendered and to determine which providers rendered services to which members. There are many other features of a utilization management system so that review nurses can answer telephones promptly, give courteous and thorough service to physicians' offices when they call, and log approved and anticipated services into an information system to track IBNR claims accurately. The group would also benefit if intramural physicians could send notification of services planned to utilization management departments by electronic mail and only interact with utilization management staff by telephone when services planned by a physician are questioned. If the group practice could communicate over a regional communications network with most other providers with which it works to care for its capitated members, those extramural physicians would benefit greatly from the ability to send notification of services planned to utilization management, avoiding the inefficiency and frustration of prior approval for services that are almost always approved.

The capitated group practice must have the ability to preprocess claims, even though the insurer that capitates the group may not want to share those data. The group needs to know about the validity, reliability, and costs of claims submitted by every provider participating in the care of the population for which it is capitated. The data need to be on-site with the group for prompt and frequent ad hoc analysis. Insurers tend to balk in making claims available to providers. They say they do not want to slow claims processing time by introducing a preprocessing (repricing) step. They add that providers are not allowed to see other providers' claims.

Under capitation, those issues are moot. Providers should insist that they preprocess claims and send them electronically to the payer. The claims are the basis for all payments to providers and for all judgments about their practice habits. Claims are receipts for services rendered. The capitated group practice needs to be able to collect, store, and retrieve for analysis all claims produced by all providers involved in the care of its patients—especially for capitated patients.

Of course, the capitated provider organization needs to keep thorough, complete, and timely financial records, including accounts payable (to participating providers), accounts receivable (from insurers and patients), general ledger, payroll, and all other financial matters. Ideally, one information system would satisfy all the information needs of the group practice. In all likelihood, however, even the most comprehensive managed care information system will not duplicate the financial management systems needed by the group practice. So the managed care system needs to be interfaced with these financial systems. All these data need to be available for retrospective analysis to improve contracting, quality of care, and marketing of the group's services.

To summarize, a group of physicians organized to care for populations of people over time under capitation needs to have access to automated information processing functions that have been the purview of health maintenance organizations and not physicians, at least until they move from fee-for-service payment to capitation. Once under capitation, they need all the information they can get on the characteristics of patients and on the services rendered to them. Managing populations of people over time, under budgets, requires an epidemiological focus on data. This is a new world for most group practices. It will bring the disciplines of informatics very much into the forefront of successful contract and population and patient management.

# Chapter 22

## Preparing for Managed Competition

Without the demands of managed competition or economic incentives to control costs, providers have little reason to invest in systematic data analysis about their patients. Information technologies in the hands of health care managers and physician executives primarily are tools for cost control. If cost control is not an important issue for them, they do not choose to use them. The rules of the game have already changed for providers where managed care dominates the medical community and will change for the entire nation under managed competition. Managed competition gives providers strong incentives to identify the costs of care and unnecessary variation in those costs, to introduce new processes of care to reduce unnecessary administrative and clinical costs, to implement practice guidelines to reduce variation in outcomes of care, and to document statistics measuring quality.

Accelerating losses of market share and profits by health care providers committed to fee-for-service payment and growing market opportunities for providers organized in integrated health care systems able to manage the care of populations of people over time speak to rapid change in the health care sector and to the importance of investing in information and communication technologies that can make integrated provider organizations perform more efficiently and effectively. The rules of competition have changed. Instead of competing through credentials and location, providers compete through measurable outcomes of care and proven technologies for networking all clinicians in the delivery system into an electronic web supporting computer-based patient records.

Consider four general categories of information technology:

- Transaction systems supporting computer-based patient records for concurrent patient care.

- Communication networks linking all locations of care to transaction systems, payers' systems, and other providers' systems.

- Enterprisewide relational databases to store data from transaction systems for retrospective continuous quality improvement studies permitting ad hoc, iterative, interactive queries from end-users.

■ Information technologies embedded in diagnostic imaging devices; radiation treatment planning systems; physiological monitors in intensive care units, operating theaters, and emergency departments; home monitoring equipment; and pacemakers, among many other emerging uses of computer technology.

One way of explaining the significance of these emerging technologies is to show their relationship to the expectations of health plan members, who have become accustomed to the benefits of these technologies in their encounters with financial services, banking, and travel and hotel industries and who expect the same kinds of services from their health care providers. For example, a hospital system in Albuquerque, New Mexico, asked managers of human resources of large corporations in their community what conveniences they want from health care delivery systems that contract to care for their employees and dependents. They summarized the responses they received into six sentences that define some of the key functional requirements of competing health care systems. By analyzing the six sentences, we can identify many information technologies required to meet the wishes of customers, and we can see the emerging importance of applied medical informatics to health care delivery systems.

*A patient—by telephone or in person at a walk-in clinic, physician's office, ambulatory diagnostic center, or hospital—can be quickly identified as an individual we have served before or as a brand new customer.*

To identify a patient accurately and consistently at any location of care within the network of health care providers requires several related computer and communications technologies that are revolutionizing other industries, especially banking and travel. To identify each patient requires an identification system that is shared by all locations of care and is understood by administrative personnel registering patients at those sites. The identification system needs to create and maintain a catalog of all past treatments at all locations so that any location can learn if a patient was treated before and how and for what purpose. Of course, patients can carry all of their medical records around with them or record accurately all the incidents of care they have had, but most patients do not want to do either.

When an electronic communications network is in place, a number of remarkable efficiencies are available to providers, and the delivery system enjoys substantial reductions in its operating costs. For instance, laboratory results produced in a hospital can be available over the network to physicians' offices in milliseconds, not the days that paper takes to travel the same distance, and can save the physician's office staff from having to call the laboratory for results. The number of telephone calls declines, and fewer clerical employees are needed to manage the remaining calls. The information is transmitted sooner, and physicians respond with other orders sooner. The velocity of clinical decision making increases.

More subtle, but more powerful, are the advisory functions that expert information systems can play with laboratory results in electronic form. A differential diagnosis can accompany the laboratory results across the network to a physician's personal computer. The differential diagnosis is produced by a network computer that scans the flow of results and occasionally recognizes a pattern for which it is programmed to comment. It makes its comments, attaches it to the laboratory results, and routes the results and the comments to the physician.

## Preparing for Managed Competition

*The patient's laboratory tests and imaging results can be transported electronically as the patient is referred within the health care delivery system, thus eliminating the need for costly and inconvenient repetition of diagnostic tests.*

One of the benefits of electronic records of patients' test results is a reduction in duplicate testing. Fewer tests are duplicated in consultants' offices if the results of the studies in primary care physicians' offices are available instantaneously over a communications network. Of course, physiological parameters change constantly, and many measurements need repeating often to follow the course of an illness. But many are repeated in two locations only because the results of the study at the first location are not available at the second location.

Laboratory test results are simple digital data to a network, as are the images produced by all diagnostic radiology equipment, with the only difference between laboratory and radiology results being the huge amounts of data required to define the images radiologists study. A serum potassium, for instance, can be represented with five bytes of information or forty bits of data (8 bits to a byte). At the speed of a 28,800 baud (bits per second) modem, which is the rate-limiting step for most wide-area networks sending data to physicians' offices, the results of a serum potassium measurement will cross over the network in less than 0.0003 seconds. On the other hand, a chest x-ray requires a minimum of 2,048 (horizontal pixels) by 2,048 (vertical pixels) by 4,096 (shades of gray per pixel) bits of data to convey its full image. With a rate-limiting modem of 28,800 baud, a full-resolution chest x-ray will cross into the physicians' personal computer in 596,523 seconds, or 6.9 days.

Obviously, no one would send a chest x-ray of so high a resolution over a network with such a slow modem. By reducing the resolution of the x-ray from diagnostic quality to "consultative" quality (1024 by 768 by 16 bits of gray scale; 1,024 by 768 by 512 bits of data) that can be presented on a standard Super VGA computer monitor, the image will pass over the 28,800 baud modem in 3.88 hours. Lowering the resolution of the x-ray still further, to 640 by 480 by 256 shades of gray, will speed up the conveyance of the image to 0.76 hours. Reducing the resolution of the image still further, to that of a standard VGA computer monitor (640 by 480 by 16 shades of gray), shortens the time to 2.8 minutes. Two and four-fifths minutes can still seem like an eternity in a busy physician's office when the computer is devoted full-time to receiving an image of an x-ray and the image will be low enough in resolution that small lung nodules, pneumothoraces, Kerley-B lines, and atelectasis may not be apparent. Nevertheless, some indication of the size of the cardiac shadow and of the location of large nodules will be apparent.

Chest x-rays and mammograms are among the highest-resolution images with which radiologists work. Much lower resolutions are required for CT scans (320 by 320 by 256 shades of gray). A single CT image would cross over that 28,800 baud modem in 15.16 minutes. Lowering the resolution to consultation quality of 320 by 320 by 16 shades of gray will reduce that time to 0.95 minutes. A CT study may still include 24 or more images, so the entire study could still take about 30 minutes to come across the network, even at low resolution. One answer to making the network useful for clinicians is to increase its speed. Modems with twice the throughput, 57,600 baud, are readily available. But greater speeds will require that we abandon the analog telephone network that forces us to use modems.

Digital networks (ISDN—Integrated Service Digital Network) are available in most urban areas now, with transmission speeds of 1,544,000 bits per second common. Speeds of hundreds of millions, and even billions, of bits per second are feasible and are available in laboratories and on special local area networks in office buildings right now. Over the next 10 years, the price of those networks will continue to plummet as our nation converts from analog to digital communications in all its work. In most office buildings, the PBX (private branch exchanges) for local telephone calling within the buildings is already digital, as are the telephones used by people in the building. Telephone companies are rapidly converting huge analog switching stations, routing millions of calls each day, to digital computers that can route many more calls at much less cost. It will not be long, less than a decade, before x-ray images near full resolution will fly from sender to recipient in a few minutes, not in days. As the transition to better technology occurs in local telephone companies, medical networks will grow in importance as a means of improving communications between providers of care to reduce inefficiencies and improve the quality of care networks can offer their members.

*Information can be viewed simultaneously by members of a quickly formed team of specialists functioning in separate locations but able to consult on the diagnosis and course of treatment for complex cases.*

In most communities, the patient or family is now the integrator of health care services, carrying x-rays and paper records from one physician to another for second opinions and consultations, waiting sometimes weeks for appointments, and often finding at the time of the appointment that the consultant knows little or nothing about the patient's condition. Consultants often consume much of appointment time perusing records from other physicians or duplicating diagnostic tests. For complicated chronic ailments, the patient or family may feel compelled to become more informed consumers of health care services, because physicians, especially subspecialists, tend to concentrate on performing procedures and all too often show little interest in managing all of the patient's complaints. Patients want the burden of being their own doctors lifted from them. They want systems of health care services that will care for them, including ensuring reliable transmission of their clinical information to specialists' offices before they visit them. Ideally, they want providers of care to come to them, rather than having to coordinate, schedule, and manage the opinions of all the providers of care themselves. They want an agency that they can trust to manage and integrate all of the health care services that they need.

Teleconferencing is commonplace now as a substitute for moving people across the globe for meetings. Video teleconferencing permits people in more than one location to speak to one another, see one another, and all see slides and other audiovisual aids used by one party in making a presentation to the others. The cost of a video teleconference using compression technologies to reduce the bandwidth required to transmit the video signals can be as low as $30 per hour, with $15,000 to $50,000 in analog video equipment at each location. Personal computers come with video cameras included. Software such as CUSeeMe allows videoconferencing between PCs over the Internet. The cost of videoconferencing is falling dramatically, as we switch from expensive analog television equipment to inexpensive digital workstations.

Considering the cost of airline travel, days away from the office, and the cost of hotel rooms and meals, today's price for video teleconferencing equipment is a bargain, and its costs are declining. Some patients, and most human resources managers of large corporations, know the benefits of teleconferencing. They will begin to expect physicians to have access by teleconferencing to radiologists for interpretation of imaging studies, to pathologists for second opinions on biopsy findings, to specialists in endoscopic surgery for counsel on endoscopic surgical procedures, to cardiologists for interpretation of unusual heart sounds and echocardiograms, and to neuroradiologists for interpretation of CT and MRI scans. The list goes on. Now, when a physician wants a consultation with another physician to guide diagnosis and treatment, the patient must travel to the consulting physician or wait for him or her to peruse the patient's medical record and images. In the future, telemedicine consultations will be scheduled more promptly, just as they often can be scheduled in a multispecialty group practice where many physicians practice in one office building. As medicine adopts teleconferencing, and the issue of who bills for the session becomes moot with capitation, the health care system will find myriad ways for teleconferencing to permit more rapid conferring between primary and consulting physicians for the sake of the patient and to preserve the velocity of care.

*Documented quality outcomes demonstrate continuous improvement in all integrated health care system locations.*

The importance to providers of documenting the outcomes of their care cannot be overemphasized. Providers must measure their value in terms of standardized outcomes of care in order to compete for the care of populations of people over time. Without the ability to collect those outcomes and report on their value in standardized ways, they will be at a decided competitive disadvantage in the managed competition marketplace.

The key to documenting quality outcomes is standardized data collection according to norms acceptable to the buyers of health care services. Standardization of all data used to study the processes and outcomes of care for patients is indispensable to an outcomes management program. Without standardized data describing patients and the services rendered to them, comparisons of outcomes and processes between different cohorts of patients may not be valid. The same rules of data collection and validation that guide the design of clinical research trials apply to clinical quality improvement and outcomes studies. The goal of these studies is to obtain information and knowledge about variations in the outcomes of care of members that can lead to improvements in the processes of care. Without valid data, the outcomes studies will be discredited, and the process improvements they suggest will never be implemented.

With standard data, comparisons between institutions may be the subject of debate; without standard data, no one will even attempt comparisons. Without measurement, there can be no systematic improvement. Without outcomes data to prove that an institution produces better outcomes than its competitors, the only thing that institution can compete on is price. Providers who can compete on measured value will earn increased market share and a premium price, just as producers of well-regarded goods and services in other industries often enjoy an economic advantage in the marketplace.

Purchasers of care do not want one uniform and bland standard of quality among providers. Most purchasers of health care services say they are willing to pay a premium for better quality, as long as they can measure it. It behooves providers to know how to measure the outcomes of care in terms of satisfaction and functional status as well as clinical events. The key to fair comparison of patients' outcomes—by physician, by specialty, by institution, by whatever cohort selected—is fair adjustment for severity of illness and case mix (together comprising risk adjustment) within the cohorts compared. Risk adjustment permits an imperfect comparison of the outcomes of care between different groups of patients. Without risk adjustment, the patients of internists who only treat diabetics may appear to have worse outcomes than do the patients of internists who perform executive physicals. Oncologists may be associated with worse outcomes than general internists, and cardiovascular surgeons at academic medical centers may seem to produce worse outcomes than do cardiovascular surgeons in community hospitals for affluent people. Risk adjustment is never perfect, but it is indispensable in leveling the playing field for providers.

The key to risk adjustment is using a methodology that is designed to predict the variation in the outcome under study. For instance, if the outcome of interest is the mortality rate for each of several community hospitals, the risk-adjustment methodology used needs to predict the variation in mortality rate as closely as possible. An adjustment methodology designed to predict variation in costs of care would not be appropriate to use to study variation in mortality rates. Parties sharing risk-adjusted data need to agree on the outcome with which to define risk and on the methodology used to predict variation in that outcome.

Health care organizations that can assign statisticians to clinical groups to build risk-adjustment models have the best chance of winning physicians' agreement. Health care organizations that purchase a vendor's product to adjust outcomes of interest for risk need to understand the limitations of whatever product they buy. The vendor's methodology is meant to explain the variation in one dependent variable, one outcome. It may be cost of care, mortality, postoperative wound infection, length of stay, a specific measure of functional status at discharge, or some measure of satisfaction at discharge. Whatever the outcome, the methodology is designed to predict variation in that outcome and not in any other outcome.

In my view, it is better to build your own models, using the data you currently collect on patients before treating them, to predict variation of outcomes of interest to you and your medical staff. A vendor's product may be appropriate, perhaps because it is required by a coalition of employers or by state government, but hire a statistician along with the software to explain as much of the model as is available to the scrutiny of users. A statistician is indispensable to any organization that is going to use its own data to do its own risk-adjustment modeling.

Most vendors of risk-adjustment systems promote the national databases they have built from data submitted by their customers. The problem with using national data sets is that observed differences between the outcomes of patients in different institutions may be attributable to differences in the ways in which data are defined or in characteristics of patients, physicians, facilities, and communities not captured in the risk-adjustment models. I counsel organizations to develop their own models or to use vendors' models that seem valid to the medical staff.

Until there is a national risk-adjustment system mandated by Congress, I suggest that health care institutions concentrate on intramural variations in outcomes of care among physicians and departments. Inside the walls of a group practice or a hospital, physicians have many more opportunities to discover ways to explain, and then reduce, variation in outcomes of care of their patients. There are too many unknown and uncertain extenuating circumstances among patients and physicians at different institutions to permit modeling of interinstitutional variation.

We do not know when a national standard data set for comparison of patients' outcomes will be established, but we do know that it will be important for organizations to have staff members who can explain and implement whatever methodology is selected. We know that report cards on the performance of provider organizations will become more common and more important to providers to help them compete on something other than price. Without health services research skills in biostatistics and epidemiology, hospitals and group practices cannot help physicians understand how their practice habits differ from those of their peers or why the outcomes of patients vary among physicians and facilities. The best investment that a health care organization can make is in staff members who know how to work with clinical and financial data for risk adjustment. Buying a proprietary software package for risk adjustment is not a good investment if staff expertise in health services research is not in place.

The buyers of health care services are asking providers to assure them that their delivery systems are giving neither too little care (from perverse incentives under capitation payment) nor too much care (from perverse incentives under fee-for-service payment). They want delivery systems to prove to them that the care they give is optimal. The buyer specifies which guidelines are important to it, and the provider will need to muster proof that patient care meets the specified guidelines. Most buyers rely on the HEDIS data set developed by NCQA.

Guidelines will play a larger role in clinical practice. Expert system software is becoming a part of most clinical transaction systems. The expert advice encoded in the logic of the systems will be available to physicians whenever they choose to use it and may appear automatically whenever a laboratory result contraindicates a certain medication or a patient's allergy contraindicates a prescribed therapeutic agent. In surgery and medicine, physicians will benefit from on-line access to current publications on the processes and outcomes of care relevant to specific patients.

Physicians are not inclined to use patient care computers directly for recording their observations about patients, entering orders for their care, or retrieving bibliographic information about their conditions, because computers are difficult for them to use. Technological changes will make computers easier to use, even engaging, and physicians will begin to use computers themselves to enter and retrieve information about their patients. When that happens, another enormous benefit of automated patient care systems will occur: Physicians will interact with computers directly, expand and improve the data collected about their patients, and take advantage of the advisory functions of those systems.

When performing procedures is remunerative and data collection is only valued for documenting and billing for those procedures, record-keeping is a necessary evil, an administrative headache, and an impediment to treating more patients. The record keeping receives short shrift. However, when physicians must care for patients under a fixed budget; when their profits depend on using health care resources effectively and efficiently; and when payers expect providers to prove that patients are improving under their care, the medical record and clinical advisory software associated with record keeping become much more valuable to physicians. Then the medical record is proof of competent care and the principal resource for continuous quality improvement, effective outcome management, and successful contract negotiations with payers.

Technologies available now, or on the horizon for widespread use in the next several years, include speaker-independent voice recognition, hand-writing recognition, and back-lit hand-held computers with touch-sensitive screens and the means of communicating over cordless infrared local area networks to patient care transaction systems. Hand-held computers with a graphical user interface and an intuitive means for physicians to enter data and orders about patients will be the physicians' most important treatment device. With them, physicians will enter observations and orders about patients and receive automated advice on differential diagnoses and therapeutic interventions to help deliver the right amounts and kinds of service to patients.

*Employers seek out integrated health care systems for custom-designed benefit packages that fully satisfy employees and that are affordable.*

This sentence, in the word "affordable," includes the first mention of the price of health care insurance. In the previous paragraph, health care services are defined by features and functions. Even in this sentence, affordable is the last word. The buyers of health care services are saying that they want features and functions, and price is there as a reminder that they can only spend so much on health care services. Providers have an opportunity to compete on features and functions, not on price alone. This should be enormously gratifying and exciting for providers and should substantiate the benefits of organizing themselves into integrated health care systems. They form an organization through which they can pool their capital, agree on the standards of information systems they share, build systems that help them compete for patients on the basis of features and functions that their customers want, and manage their costs successfully.

Custom-designed benefit packages appeal to employers and employees because they can have just the health care benefits they want, with a provider network, covered services, and rules about eligibility and cost-sharing and utilization management customized for them. Unfortunately, primary care physicians must deal with a unique plan for each insurer with which they sign a contract. The complexity of dealing with 30, or more, different lists of participating providers, and as many sets of guidelines for utilization management, prior approval, and collection of copayments, has become an enormous financial burden to primary care offices. Computer technology permits physicians' offices to access current eligibility and benefits information about patients when they appear in their offices and to send claims electronically after office visits.

Under managed competition, health care delivery systems contract directly with large employers or the purchasing agents of smaller employers for the capitated care of populations of people over time. Providers either own an HMO or contract with a large insurer that "owns" the delivery system. When providers and purchasers are organized, small indemnity insurance companies and insurance brokers disappear.

How do computers promote these trends? Once information and communication technologies are standardized among all providers and are used by them for their patients, providers can perform their work far more efficiently and effectively, with far better information, than they ever could before. The character and the economics of the care change. The quality of care improves while costs moderate. The providers transform themselves into something entirely new, an integrated health care delivery system with a functioning nervous system that is made of standardized transaction, communication, and decision support systems.

## Conclusion

The functional requirement of quickly identifying each patient at every possible location of care defines the need for an electronic communication system linking all the locations of care; computer equipment at each location that clerks, nurses, and physicians know how to use; and a master person indexing (MPI) system so that people at each location know how to identify uniquely each person who requests care. Beneficiaries will carry identification cards, and, over a communication network, providers will access not only the MPI for each beneficiary but also summary data from a computer-based patient record of past health care visits, procedures, diagnoses, medications, and allergies.

The beneficiary identification card gives providers access to the MPI over the network and to a summary medical record for each patient. For there to be a summary computer-based patient record (CPR) on each beneficiary, the delivery system must have interfaces between clinical transaction systems at locations of care and the database that serves as the CPR. Interfaces are computer programs that translate the data fields, and their formats, into the format of the CPR. The more laboratory and radiology transaction systems, the more interfaces that must be created, at costs of $50,000 or more each.

Telemedicine has proved cost-effective in many countries and in many settings for many different kinds of patients. A limitation to the adoption of telemedicine has been the reluctance of insurers to pay physicians for telemedicine consultations. They require a "face-to-face" visit between physician and patient. Once patients are enrolled in systems and providers have responsibility for clinical care and its costs, the issue of billing will be moot, and the efficiency of telemedicine increases its uses.

Providers use information technologies to document their outcomes of care and continuously improve their work. Buyers of health care services require provider organizations to compete for the care of their beneficiaries on the basis of outcomes. Providers share a standardized vocabulary for defining procedures and diagnoses, as well as patients' satisfaction and outcomes. Their transaction systems use the same standardized vocabulary, and interfaces between transaction systems and the communications network allow summary information about patients' diagnoses, procedures, results, satisfaction, and functional status to flow electronically, without duplicate data entry, into a computer-based patient record that also resides on the network. The CPR depends on a relational database for retrospective analysis, with powerful software tools to make simple the asking of ad hoc queries to identify opportunities for quality improvement in the processes of care. Without these analytical capabilities, providers have a difficult time competing for patients at any price.

Providers need a means of placing standard treatment guidelines at the fingertips of clinicians. Books of guidelines do not suffice. Over the communication network, physicians obtain current guidelines about diagnostic work-ups, differential diagnoses, and treatment plans based on the unique characteristics of their patients. Guidelines are broad enough to apply to more than one patient but refined enough to be useful to physicians with specific patients in mind. The guidelines are easy to update and readily available over the network. Clinical transaction systems bring up guidelines automatically when some constellation of signs, symptoms, and laboratory results leads a physician to request one.

Customers want a variety of health care benefit plans, and they want providers to deal with them efficiently. Customers want providers organized to deal with them directly, not necessarily through an insurance intermediary. Customers want all these features at a price they can afford, but not necessarily the price of the cheapest health insurance program. Customers want providers to compete on services and value rather than on price alone. Physicians and hospitals that do not join integrated delivery systems of their own creation, and choose instead to contract with insurers, find themselves forced to compete on price with other providers.

Information technologies are the glue that hold integrated health care systems together and that permit distribution of patients' records; efficient coordination of services; and promulgation of guidelines to participating physicians, allied health professionals, and managers in multiple locations of care. Providers who have invested in those technologies and have incorporated them into their delivery of care to patients find themselves more attractive to purchasers of health care services than do providers who have not done so.

# Chapter 23

# New Governance for a New Era: Issues and Challenges for Integrating Systems

In chapter 19, I identified and briefly described five factors that I believe will define an integrated system's ability to compete successfully in the new marketplace for health care services that is now unfolding. I want to expand on my earlier discussion and add several factors.

**Attract and Retain Physicians**
Without physicians, the integrated delivery system (IDS) will not win contracts with employers, insurers, or health plans and will not take care of patients. The IDS cannot grow any faster than it can acquire physicians to treat patients. The IDS can do many things to attract physicians into its organization. Most physicians complete training with considerable debt to colleges and medical schools they attended. Most physicians look for a safe way to start seeing patients, without taking on more debt and risk to start a solo practice. The IDS can reduce a new physician's practice costs by including him or her in an existing group practice, giving him or her a salary with bonus for treating more patients than expected, and making available state-of-the-art information systems that he or she may have used in training but could not afford were he or she to start practice alone. The benefits of group practice—guaranteed minimum income, insulation from administrative hassles, camaraderie with partner physicians, access to sophisticated practice managers, more leverage in managed care contracting, ability to participate in capitated contracts with relatively little personal financial risk, sense of security and future prospects for practice growth, continuing clinical education, and access to advanced information systems, including computer-based patient records and telecommunication networks linking physicians' offices and facilities, to name a few benefits—will appear increasingly more persuasive to physicians.

**Establish Standards**
A loose consortium of facilities that call themselves collectively an integrated delivery system deceives itself. Information processing and distribution are standardized throughout a real integrated system. Information systems and data dictionaries are standardized; business processes are standardized; and senior managers, physicians, and boards of directors of the various operating units cede some of their authority to senior managers, physicians, and board of directors of the parent organization.

During the transition from fee-for-service to capitation, member organizations of IDSs suffer considerable ambivalence, recognizing the theoretical value of standardized ways of collecting, storing, communicating, retrieving, and analyzing data about the services they render and the outcomes of their patients, but yearning for the independence to establish whatever management and clinical practices make the most sense to them, with whatever information and communication systems appeal most to them. They choose to ignore the enormous boon to any economy that happens when standards emerge, and they rationalize ignoring standards for practice guidelines and automated information systems because their needs are different from, and more urgent than, those of any other operating unit of the so-called IDS.

Those who govern the IDS must force independent operating units to adhere to standards where standards will allow the entire system to operate more effectively and efficiently. Standards are indispensable for integration of the electronic flow of information about health plan members and patients within the system. They are essential if data about members and patients are to be collected in relational databases for systematic, retrospective analysis that can lead to opportunities for steady practice improvement.

## Integrate Care

We cannot integrate care without integrating information about the members and patients we serve and about the health care services we produce. Care is organized, and integrated, by the sharing of information. The home health agency needs to know about the diagnoses and treatments given to patients in hospital. Subspecialists need to know what primary care physicians want them to do in their consultations. Clinicians need to know the results of diagnostic studies performed in radiology centers and laboratories. Management needs to know about the services provided and the resources consumed throughout the organization and about yet unmet needs of patients, members, and providers if they are to allocate capital effectively and efficiently.

Integrating care reduces unnecessary duplication of diagnostic tests, repetition of treatments that have been ineffectual in the past, and the time required for consultants to learn about the past medical histories of patients on whom they are consulting.

Integrating care also helps to standardize care and the data collected about care, which greatly enhances opportunities for retrospective studies to reveal opportunities for quality improvement. If every physician uses his or her own idiosyncratic style in treating every patient, reliable data for clinical research will be hard to come by and relatively useless to study. But if clinicians in the IDS collect data about their patients and introduce treatments in a standardized way consistent with good clinical research discipline, observations made on patients' outcomes can be enormously informative to the IDS and help both clinicians and managers improve the processes of care for members and patients.

Integrating care includes instituting standard means of collecting and storing data about members and patients; standardizing contracting so that every operating unit of the IDS works under a standard contract with any given payer; cultivating a standard clinical and managerial culture that includes all providers and managers of facilities; standardizing the data dictionary of electronic transaction systems so that procedure costs, formularies, and laboratory reports have the same consistent terms throughout the organization; and vesting in an information systems council for the IDS the power to dictate to operating units that they must adhere to standards set by the organization for information and communication systems. Standardization of data and automation of data and information processing are key characteristics of growing, consolidating, competitive industries.

## Conserve Capital

No business can afford to squander capital for long. Since the 1960s, when generous indemnity health insurance was made available to most Americans, health care providers have enjoyed the ability to pass along their operating costs to consumers of their services (patients and insurers) and thereby guarantee profits year in and year out. Consequently, health care costs have risen faster than general inflation every year, until recently. As delivery systems compete for patients more aggressively and as insurers reduce the fees they pay providers, IDSs will need to husband their capital carefully. They will have major demands for capital in the near future, among them to recruit and retain physicians, to establish health plans and managed care insurance products, and to modernize their information and communication systems.

Most hospitals are not-for-profit and many IDSs are not-for-profit, so the capital they obtain comes from savings and debt. As for-profit managed care organizations grow and capture a larger share of the insurance market (currently 69 percent of health plans, covering 55 percent of enrollees, are for-profit), provider-sponsored IDSs will need all the sources of capital at their disposal. They don't pay taxes, but they also don't have access to equity capital. They need to concentrate on efficient operations and on saving money for that rainy day that may be just around the corner.

## Grow Strategically

Strategic growth is a euphemism for smart growth, not the growth all too often seen among IDSs that have emerged from regional hospital systems that grew horizontally, acquiring community hospitals whose administrators were good buddies of the senior executives of the hospital-based IDS. Hospitals had capital to waste. They don't any longer, as more care is delivered outside the hospital. Hospitals need to save their money for alliances with physicians and for health plans and information systems. Technology is reducing the value of hospitals as warehouses of beds. The increasing importance of efficient health care processes is raising the value to IDSs of alliances with physicians committed to their financial success and growth. The IDS needs the capital to invest in information and communication systems that will enhance the efficiency of practice for physicians and in health plans that will help physicians market their services more successfully.

Strategic growth means growing into business activities not commonly associated with hospitals—health plans, group practices, and networks of participating physicians. The cultural changes associated with this shift are difficult for many hospital administrators and board members to accomplish. They wish they could go on forever acquiring and managing hospitals and dealing with hospital people. But they can't. They need detailed, long-range strategic plans that say more than, "Do good, bill for all, and keep everybody happy." They need to specify how, and in what ventures, they will invest their capital, even if those statements alienate portions of the medical staff or other community leaders and reduce the significance of the hospital in the larger IDS.

## Control Costs

Controlling costs of health care services is the only means of generating revenue in excess of costs (profits) that is available to providers and IDSs that receive most of their income from capitation. Group- and staff-model HMOs have lived with this reality for decades, but now IDSs emerging from regional hospital systems receive most of their revenue, and most of their profits, from managed care contracts. In fact, the parts of those organizations that are growing most quickly are their home health agencies and their health plans, and the health plans return income to the provider portions of the organizations with capitation. Primary care capitation has become common in most urban areas, and group practices are becoming accustomed to carve-outs and fixed price contracts more quickly than hospitals. Controlling variable costs means controlling the costs and volume of supplies and services rendered to patients. Controlling fixed costs means controlling the costs of capital, insurance, and other business associated with the location of services rendered and the overhead of the organization providing those services.

In the long run, all costs are variable and can be changed. In the short run of one year or less, many costs appear to be fixed. Most of the costs of care are direct clinical costs. Consequently, systematic clinical data analysis for quality improvement studies may reveal many opportunities to reduce clinical costs. For most common ailments, there is a wide variation in the processes of care used by clinicians, with attendant wide variation in the costs of that care, without nearly as dramatic variation in clinical outcomes and functional status of patients after treatment. Clinical data must be adjusted for patients' probability of outcomes before treatment. Once such an adjustment is made, the efficiency and effectiveness of clinicians' practice habits can be compared.

Risk adjustment is not a perfect science, but useful observations can still be made with less than perfect data. Analytical staff skilled in risk adjustment, and familiar with clinical practice, select the risk-adjustment methods to which patients' data are subjected and obtain approval for the methods used before the data at hand are adjusted for the prior probability of the outcome in question. After a risk-adjustment methodology is accepted by clinicians, they are more likely to accept the adjusted results as valid and to participate in quality improvement programs based on the results of the studies.

## Process Information Well

Proficiency in processing information is a goal to which all organizations aspire. They all strive to move information from place to place in the organization as quickly and accurately as possible in order to reduce their operating costs and improve services to customers. In integrated delivery systems, information proficiency implies successful movement of administrative and clinical information about patients. Most health care organizations invest resources in automation of administrative information first, because processing claims accurately and quickly reduces the age and total value of funds in their accounts receivable. Automation helps to capture more charges than does manual processing of services and to reduce the labor costs of collecting, storing, retrieving, communicating, and managing data about charges.

Now, many insurers demand that claims from providers, especially hospitals, be submitted electronically to expedite payment and reduce the costs to insurers of manual entry of claims into their claims processing systems. Automation of clinical information is common in clinical laboratories and is becoming common in radiology departments. Results are distributed to clinicians sooner, and automation allows for more complete accounting of services rendered to patients, so providers can produce more accurate, and larger, bills for services rendered. Automation of medical records is not common except where transcription is performed by word processing systems. In such systems, text transcribed from clinicians' dictation is moved electronically from the word processing system into a patient care information system that clinicians use to retrieve clinical results from workstations on the nursing units of hospitals and in the offices of group practices.

There are not yet strong economic incentives for providers to invest in automated medical record systems for clinicians to use in their daily care of patients. Technologies for data collection are not efficient enough for physicians to abandon pen and paper, or dictation, to capture their clinical observations about patients. Nevertheless, the day is dawning when clinicians will prefer workstations with voice recognition for entering their clinical observations about patients and hand-held, back-lit, portable computers to retrieve results and enter orders. That day must be preceded by considerable investment in capital and new governance initiatives among the operating units of IDSs.

For instance, before a computer-based patient record can be shared electronically among the many locations of care in an IDS, the locations must have adopted a master person index (standardized patient identification) and have given patients identification and medical record numbers with a common methodology. The operating units must share a common data dictionary, so that data elements in the electronic records mean the same thing in every facility. The transaction systems used in the various operating units need to have the same look and feel so that clinicians moving from one facility to another can use the computer-based patient record wherever they go. The data collected by these standardized transaction systems should be copied to a relational data repository (data warehouse) where clinicians and managers can access them easily to compare the processes and outcomes of care of the various operating units, looking for variation in outcomes that suggest opportunities for quality improvement. The leaders of the organization need instruction in medical informatics, so they know the implications of these automated information systems and how to analyze data to improve the organization's processes and outcomes of care.

In the near future, most health care organizations, including IDSs, will acquire two computer-based patient record technologies—one for on-line transaction processing (OLTP) of physicians' orders and laboratory results, scheduling, and medical records maintenance, and the other for on-line analytical processing (OLAP), with a data model and software tools meant to make retrospective health services and clinical research as efficient and comprehensive as possible. The OLTP system uses a normalized relational database designed for rapid (1-2 second) response times for every change of screen for hundreds, if not thousands, of simultaneous users. The OLAP system uses a denormalized relational database of relatively few relational tables and software designed to make iterative, ad hoc data analysis efficient from users' point of view. The OLAP system is designed to support epidemiology and public health studies, which, in turn, form the intellectual basis of continuous clinical quality improvement studies.

As information flows, so goes the organization. If information does not flow smoothly from the central part of the organization to a peripheral operating unit, such as a group practice or a hospital, the peripheral unit is not an integral part of the organization. If each operating unit (hospital, group practice, HMO, home health agency, urgent care center) maintains its own financial and clinical information systems, and information is conveyed between operating units on paper, the organization probably does not behave like an integrated system. Rather, it behaves like a loose confederation of otherwise independent entities. On the other hand, if operating units have invested the time and effort and capital to standardize their operations and their information systems, information flows from one operating unit to another seamlessly, clinicians in one location can obtain computer-based patient records of patients treated in any other location, and financial transactions are integrated so that patients paying fee for service receive one integrated bill for all services (facility fees and professional fees) from all providers, the governing body of the organization has created a true integrated delivery system.

Unfortunately, most organizations that claim to be integrated delivery systems are not integrated at all when it comes to the flow of information between their various locations and operating units. Until clinical care of patients is perceived to be a continuum over all primary care physicians, subspecialists, ancillary services, and facilities of the organization, the organization will appear to be a collection of independent practitioners organized to produce procedures at single points in time and not to manage the welfare of a population of patients over time in the most efficient and effective manner possible. The latter organization is our stated goal, but we persist in protecting our older models of organization. We are changing, slowly. Information technologies we could use to expedite the transformation of our organizations to integrated delivery systems are improving much faster than are our habits of governance and organization.

# Section IV

## Implications for Providers and Provider Organizations

# Chapter 24
## Changes and Choices for Physicians

A prudent buyer is a strong force for value in health care purchases. Health care is complicated and uncertain, and the buyer does not have a lot of information to guide decisions. Fifty years ago, very little in medicine was discretionary, but now physicians have a large number of choices, and it isn't always clear which choice is best. It is easier to assess the necessity of the care in retrospect than at the time of delivery.

Employers cannot assume that the physician is greedy or doing something bad if "unnecessary" services are delivered. "Unnecessary" is in the eye of the beholder. The demands of the purchaser or the patient matter. Whether a person tolerates a knee injury and works through the healing process or chooses a surgical intervention is up to the person as much as to the doctor.

**Market Incentives Drive Health Care**
Health care is financed in the same way we finance the manufacture of many products, necessary or not. When buying personal computers, most people purchase more components than they need. We all celebrate this economic model in the United States, because it produces a wide variety of high-quality goods and services and generates jobs. Yet the same economic model in health care leads to "unnecessary" services.

With fee-for-service and indemnity insurance, we get what we pay for. Cost-based, fee-for-service medicine, developed in the 1940s by Blue Cross and Blue Shield in Texas, increased access to the latest technology and specialized physicians. It is a system of financing health care that removes economic impediments to people benefiting from the latest technology. There are no economic incentives for hospitals and physicians to save the community money by rejecting technology, only to see their competitor buy the technology, do the procedures, and bring in the revenue.

Physicians respond to economic incentives in the marketplace. All the financial incentives for physicians favor doing procedures. Compared with doctors who do laparoscopic cholecystectomies, arthroscopies, colonoscopies, cardiac surgery, and neurosurgery, primary care physicians earn next to nothing. PCPs are expected to convince people to change poor personal health habits, which account for about half of all the costs of health care. It may take numerous office visits to the primary care physician to help a three-pack-a-day smoker quit. But the PCP earns only a small fraction of what a cardiologist earns for catheterizing a smoker's coronary arteries.

Young physicians with a debt burden of more than $100,000 tend to pick surgical or medical specialties that enable them to make the most money. An internist is paid $50 to $75 an hour to help patients lose weight and stop smoking; a cardiologist earns thousands of dollars for every cardiac catheterization.

Newer procedures usually are more remunerative than the ones they replace, helping to drive the proliferation of new techniques. Once an insurer sets a price for a procedure, the price usually tends to increase with inflation, but new procedures are priced at a higher level than the ones they replace.

As a result, the benefits of economies of scale and efficient production have not been passed on to health care purchasers. Over a decade, ophthalmologists expanded their capability to do cataract extractions from 1 to 10 per day. However, the price of a cataract extraction continued to go up at a rate equal to or greater than inflation. Ophthalmologists saw their annual incomes go from $200,000 to $800,000.

Diseases are being diagnosed earlier and treated more effectively, but there is a catch. As the pain and difficulty of treatment declines, the number of patients increases. More orthopedic surgery is being done than ever before. One can debate whether the proportion of orthopedic surgical cases is increasing unnecessarily or not, but it is clear that, as the pain of such surgery declines and more people run and stay fit, the demand for procedures is growing. We know more and we can do more. The problem is, when should we stop? Patients do not want to stop. Often, they want more care than the doctor is willing to provide.

Providers respond to market pressures. The United States has the highest nominal costs for health care per capita. The United States also has, by far, the shortest length of stay for hospital care. Hospitals have been under market pressure to lower length of stay for two decades. The result has been pushing a lot of indirect costs quite appropriately out to the employer, the employee, home health care, and a lot of other services. The marketplace has responded with the development of outpatient technologies. Surgery can now be done on an outpatient basis that wasn't dreamed of 5 and 10 years ago. In the health care cost equation, however, it is volume and proliferation of services that are driving cost and quality, not length of stay in hospitals.

## The Provider Perspective
Providers, especially physicians, overwhelmingly feel a loss of control. They feel badgered by utilization review firms and bombarded by varying terms and conditions in their contracts with payers. They hear they must sign up for a health plan or lose patients to a competitor next door. Physicians sense that either hospitals or insurers are going to own them.

Meanwhile, primary care physicians and some specialists are seeing their practice overhead reach 75 percent of net revenue, versus 50 percent or less 10 years ago. Yet, the prices for primary care services have not gone up much at all. The United States has more hospital administrators than any nation on earth because of managed care issues and massive administrative burdens.

# Changes and Choices for Physicians

Providers don't trust insurers, who they believe are trying to shift much of the financial risk of care to them. Malpractice premiums may amount to only one to two percent of total health care spending, but they are a big issue, particularly if a physician is trying to dissuade a patient from doing something he or she read about in a magazine. Providers view malpractice litigation as a way to redistribute income in our society to people who have had unfortunate events, whether the doctor was negligent or not.

To keep up with every new development, a doctor would have to read 300 journals a day. No industry on earth generates the kind of research and reporting that medicine does. New drugs come out every day. Physicians cannot keep up. Pharmaceutical houses do a service by providing physicians with detailed information and a disservice by not telling doctors that generic medications are usually as good as brand-named products.

Although they are seeing more pressure from managed care, physicians don't want to change. Nor do hospitals. Medicine is still a wonderful profession. Although many physicians wish that insurers would pay generous fee-for-service payments and leave them alone, they know that the market is not going to grant this wish and that they are going to have to change their ways.

Providers are grudgingly holding meetings to seek solutions. Many physicians accept that they are going to be practicing in organized care systems. Some are even convinced this may actually be better than the old system because they will not have to worry as much about administration.

## An Organized System of Care

Providers are interested in moving to a system of "organized care," where providers govern themselves to deliver cost-effective care. This is not the same as managed care as we know it today. In organized systems of care, providers will get away from the micromanagement and paperwork of managed care.

Providers are recognizing the need to aggregate into larger medical firms. Managed care contracting requires integrated delivery systems just to handle the contracts. No single physician or hospital can take care of 100,000 people. Multiple locations, specialties, and facilities are needed. Sutter, a multihospital system in northern California, received no revenue from physician-hospital organizations four years ago. Now more than a billion dollars, one-half of its revenue, flows through its physician-hospital organizations.

Provider organizations are beginning to put resources into information technologies that the banking and travel industries invested in 20 years ago. Expenditures for information systems are likely to triple in the next few years. The outcome will be computer-based patient records with which medical care can be managed more effectively. For example, Kaiser has announced a 2.6 billion dollar investment in developing computer-based patient records for northern California.

You cannot have an organized care system without three fundamental components, which cost a lot of money:

- **Standardized data collection.** Increasingly, performance data need to be collected with insurers and employers in mind. The data must support quality management efforts and demonstrate to payer and patients that they are receiving efficient, effective medicine. Employers are helping the process by demanding data. Although there are some national standards emerging (e.g., Short Form 36 for functional status measurement, the Uniform Clinical Data Set for hospital care, HEDIS for health plans), we do not yet have data standards to identify patients, members, and providers reliably. The HIPAA of 1996 may give us data standards for basic identification of each American and standards for electronic communication of basic administrative data between provider and payer.

- **Telecommunications networks.** Such networks link all of the transaction systems that collect data. Telemedicine is going to transform medical practice. It will enable the delivery of care right to the home via the same technology being used by cable TV and telephone companies. More than 200 major trials of telemedicine are going on around the United States. Check out the Telemedicine Information Exchange to get all the latest information about telemedicine (http://tie.telemed.org).

- **Data warehouses** for health services research help physicians understand their clinical practice habits over time. Information systems will also provide important support. Micromanaging doctors at the bedside is inefficient because so many extenuating circumstances surround medical care. Every patient is different, and every patient's circumstances are different. Doctors have to deal with those differences. But, for similar types of patients, one would expect physicians' practices to be similar. Wide variation in practice habits warrants attention.

## What Physicians Want

Physicians do not unanimously agree on what needs to be done in the current tumultuous market for health care services, but a number of trends are evident:

### Group Practices

Since 1980, the number of physicians entering group practice has grown faster than the number of physicians entering practice. The net effect is that every physician finishing training is going into a group. Salaried employment for physicians, managed care contracting, and participation in health maintenance organizations (HMOs) and capitation are all growing. The American College of Physician Executives, which helps physicians understand the business aspects of what they do, represents the fastest growing specialty of medicine. Still, the number of applicants to medical school is increasing, at a rate of as much as 10 percent a year over the past five years.

### Contracts With Employers

Proactive physicians are seeking to form organized systems of care to contract directly with employers and insurers. They would appreciate collaborating with employers and insurers to develop benefit plans that do not interfere with the provision of necessary and cost-effective care. A case in point is home care. Often, medical services that could be delivered in the home aren't paid for if they are delivered in the home. For payment, the services must be delivered in the hospital. Physicians understand the processes of medicine better than anyone else, and they want to bring that talent to a partnership with payers, to design a more rational health care system.

## Quality of Care

Physicians want to be able to compete on quality, and they are coming to accept that the value of what they do is going to be determined by analyzing data on outcomes and habits over time. In general, physicians don't receive back from insurers or employers summary or comparative data with which to assess the quality of their practices. With retrospective data, an organized system of care can get a physician's attention and change his or her behavior. The British Health Service produced many studies in the past 10 years that show physicians' practice habits and outcomes of care for their patients improve when they receive valid profiling data.*

## Changing Employee Expectations

Providers want employers to work with them to change the biases and the expectations of employees. Providers don't want to accept capitation and then have employees expect fee for service, with all of the inefficiencies that fee for service may bring. Patients end up disliking providers who tell them they don't need to consume as many health care services as they may want.

## Employer Challenges

The first challenge for employers is to become more prudent purchasers. Clearly, having physicians in the ranks of senior management helps.

Second, they must prepare employees to prevent ailments. From the provider's perspective, employers are too timid in trying to change their employees' habits. Employers need to teach employees about prevention as much as the medical professional needs to tell them about it. Clearly, the greatest savings come from preventing disease, not in treating it.

Third, employers ought to endorse information systems that allow a physician to better manage patient care. Eventually, technology will enable physicians to talk to employees at home in two-way teleconferencing rather than force those employees to go to a doctor's office or an emergency department.

Fourth, employers need to focus on the total costs, both direct and indirect, of illness and injury. Capitation can minimize provider costs, but it does not necessarily minimize payer costs. For the health plan, hospitals, procedural physicians, and home health care are all cost centers. Lost time from work is an additional cost to the employer but not to the health plan. Providers can help employers get people back to work as soon as possible at the lowest total cost. They understand the relationship between health and health care, cost control, and cost effectiveness.

Finally, employers need to understand that they will get what they pay for. Minimizing capitation payments only serves to squeeze providers, who respond by protecting themselves financially. Providers have the most knowledge of the health care process. It is better to match capitation with outcomes, such as functional status, satisfaction, and costs.

---

\* Mugford, M., and others. "Effects of Feedback on Information on Clinical Practice—A Review," *BMJ* 303(6799):398-402, Aug. 17, 1991.

Standardization and provider cooperation lead to better care. Costs of care are lower in multispecialty group practice. An unstructured fee-for-service system in which every provider is a separate profit center is not managed care. To manage the delivery of necessary and appropriate health care services under a budget, an organized delivery system is necessary.

# Chapter 25
## Physician Profiling

We are accustomed to profiling professional athletes. We measure the performances of our athletes on the field completely. We use carefully compiled statistics to select them for our teams, label the best of them as all-stars, calculate their incomes, rank their accomplishments for posterity, admit them to various halls of fame, and plot their gradual senescence to retirement. We argue about who was the best batter with lifetime batting and slugging averages; runs batted in; and counts of singles, doubles, triples, and home runs. We debate about the best professional running back with measurements of average yards per carry, average carries per game, number of touchdowns, and success of the teams on which he played. We rank professional hockey forwards by their average goals and assists per game, their total goals and assists, and the records of their teams in competition for division titles and the Stanley Cup.

How are litigators measured? Clearly, by the proportion of cases they litigate to victory for their clients and by the income they generate for their firms. Some attorneys are measured by the number of articles they publish in legal journals and by the number of clients they bring to their firms. Management consultants and accountants are measured in a similar way. Legal and accounting firms face increasing competition, as more of their customers negotiate fixed price contracts. How are the partners responsible for those fixed revenue accounts evaluated? Their firms know what they negotiated as fees and can estimate the costs of servicing those contracts. The partners are evaluated on the basis of the profits (or losses) of their firms in servicing those accounts. Engineering and advertising firms have more experience with fixed price contracts. They routinely propose fixed price contracts to their potential customers in soliciting business. The partners who craft those proposals are measured by the business they generate and by the profits (or losses) their firms incur in meeting their obligations under those contracts.

How are movie directors measured? By the profits (or losses) the movies they direct generate. Behind the profits (or losses) are the skills of the director to capture footage that will interest enough people to pay money to see the film so that the revenue generated by the movie exceeds the expenses of making it. Of course, the director has to be able to motivate people; plan complex logistics of casting, staging, and film production; and control budgets. But his or her performance is defined by the profits (or losses) of the films he or she directs.

Consider the managers of mutual funds. How are they evaluated by their employers? By the growth of their mutual funds, which, in turn, is directly related to the total annual financial return of their funds and the performance of their funds in bull and bear markets. There are many details that go into successful selection of financial goods—stocks and bonds—for mutual funds, but the measures of success are growth and annual financial return of the fund.

## Profiles of Professionals Are Measures of Their Outcomes

There is one common characteristic of runs batted in, slugging averages, goals and assists per game, free throw percentages, points and assists per game, numbers of new customers per year, total revenue produced per year, ratio of revenue to cost of films, and total annual return of a mutual fund. They are all measures of the key outcomes of the persons producing them. The better those outcomes, the more valuable are the persons producing them.

The education, experience, training, and hard work that went into producing those outcomes do not matter in the marketplace. The customer has no interest in paying for the processes used to produce movies, contracts, engagements, and annual returns. The customer wants and pays for outcomes. We measure golfers by the number of tournaments they have won. We count the basketball player's assists, points, blocked shots, steals, and free throws made per game. All the training that goes into an athlete we take for granted. We know basketball, football, baseball, and hockey players, golfers, investment managers, corporate executives, engineers, lawyers, and movie directors have invested decades of hard work to perfect their skills in the marketplace, and we may enjoy watching them perform their work, but we determine their incomes and bonuses, and their eligibility for accolades, by their outcomes.

Competition and commerce depend on standardized measures of the goods and services traded. An owner of a professional football team will insist on knowing the measures of a prospective quarterback's performance in college and will pay more for one with a higher pass completion average, larger number of yards covered on offense per game, and higher percentage of games won than he will for a quarterback with lower scores on those key outcomes, provided those outcomes are adjusted for the competition the quarterback's team faced.

When you consider buying stocks or bonds, you rely on generally accepted accounting principles (GAAP) to define the financial performance of the corporation whose financial assets you may purchase. The marketplace for stocks and bonds utterly depends on trust that the profits and losses, net income, and assets and liabilities of all corporations allowed to sell such assets are calculated in the same way. We measure the relative value of stocks by their price-to-earnings (P/E) ratios and their current prices per share. The price is determined in the marketplace. Earnings are determined by accountants and independent auditors, who define earnings as the excess of all revenue after all expenses have been paid. Earnings depend on an accurate, and standard, accounting of revenue and expense. How can you compare the P/E ratio of the common stocks of two corporations if the E is determined in a different way for each firm?

Now, consider the practice of medicine. Medicine may be more difficult to practice than any of these other professions. Medicine may require more intellectual talent and longer years of training than these other professions. Medicine may include more process variables and more outcomes of importance, and those outcomes may be harder to measure. Nevertheless, we are learning to measure the processes and outcomes of medicine every day. Learning to measure the processes will help us codify them into practice guidelines. Learning the outcomes will allow us to define the performance, and determine the market value, of providers and health plans.

The concentration on outcomes in medicine coincides with medicine's maturation into a business in which contracts between purchasers of care (employers and insurers) and delivery systems of providers determine which providers treat which patients. The outcomes movement in medicine also coincides with our emerging ability to measure and standardize the processes and outcomes of medical care. We have standardized nomenclatures for diagnoses and procedures (CPT-4 and ICD9-CM), for patients' functional status (Short Form-36), for physicians' findings on examinations before and after surgery (TyPE scales), and for health risk (health risk appraisals). We have inexpensive means of storing all those data in electronic form, in relational databases on personal computers, to permit rapid analysis of clinical and financial data. We have learned how to adjust for the prior probabilities of specific outcomes in patients—before clinicians' treatments increase the likelihood of good outcomes and reduce the probability of undesirable outcomes.

## Profiling Medical Professionals and Their Firms

Competition and commerce have come to medicine. Cost-based indemnity insurance is less available every day. Providers' customers are health insurers that want to purchase health care services for their beneficiaries from providers willing to accept some, or all, of the financial risk for the care of those defined populations. Providers are aggregating into competing delivery systems, most of them defined by large insurers that have organized HMOs and PPOs that contract with individual hospitals and physicians. But some organizations of providers contract directly with employers. Employers want the means to compare the virtues of various health care delivery systems that they may offer to their beneficiaries, considering outcomes in addition to premium price.

In the absence of differentiating outcomes among health plans, most employers select health plans (and their networks of providers) on the basis of premium price. But some beneficiaries successfully sue for damages when health care insurers and employers restrict their access to medical care to specific delivery systems that deliver inadequate care. Not all delivery systems are alike. Characteristics other than price are important to define the "quality" of a health care delivery system. Employers and insurers want to measure those characteristics. Providers who want to earn more money for better work will want those characteristics measured.

The era of profiling hospitals arrived in the 1980s, when the Health Care Financing Administration began paying hospitals fixed case rates for Medicare patients. In turn, hospitals began to study the practice habits of physicians, because their orders for services for Medicare inpatients determined whether or not the hospitals profited from the care they delivered. The profiling was limited to inpatients, and most of the profiling was kept from the purview of the physicians profiled.

Public comparisons of outcomes were limited to hospitals after states began collecting standardized outcomes measures of inpatients in the 1980s. Pennsylvania mandates that medical records of all inpatients be abstracted by the proprietary MedisGroups methodology from MediQual. California and New York require hospitals to report on inpatient admissions using the standard UB-92 data set but risk-adjust those data by proprietary methodologies developed by each state. Virginia requires the same data collection from hospitals but uses another commercial methodology for risk adjustment.

More than 40 states now collect a limited, standardized data set on all patients treated in hospitals. While most states collect the uniform billing abstract (UB-92) for every inpatient—which includes up to nine diagnosis codes and six procedure codes, birth date, admission date, discharge data, and discharge status of every patient—no state collects detailed data from outpatient visits, excluding claims data from Medicaid. States are not creating large databases of claims from inpatient and outpatient services with which to profile physicians' practice habits over episodes of illness. Efforts to profile physicians' practice habits over episodes of illness are limited to insurers with large claims databases. Insurers are beginning to use those databases to invite individual physicians and group practices for their "select" PPO networks, meant to replace their open preferred provider panels that include most providers in any given community.

## Economic Credentialing

Hospitals use the discharge abstract (UB-92) to profile physicians' practice habits for economic credentialing, deciding, in a few well-documented cases that have led to litigation, that certain clinicians do not warrant admitting privileges because their practice habits adversely affect the economic performance of the hospital. A substantial number of legal cases appear to have established a clear precedent in favor of a hospital's right to withhold admitting privileges on the basis of economic issues. In the absence of discrimination based on age, race, sex, ethnic background, or creed of a physician, hospitals may apply economic credentialing to all physicians and set arbitrary standards that may lead the hospital to withhold admitting privileges from some physicians.

Physicians have argued in court that such behavior violates antitrust statutes, but the courts have found that physicians are sellers of services to patients (and hospitals) and not consumers of hospital services. Antitrust statutes are meant to protect consumers. They do not apply in most situations of loss of admitting privileges. Courts have determined that the board of directors of a hospital has ultimate authority over the credentialing process and may unilaterally rule against the interests of a member of the medical staff. In fact, in spite of the publicity given to economic credentialing, very few physicians lose their admitting privileges at hospitals, because every physician represents potential fee-for-service income to each hospital where he or she has admitting privileges. Physicians who do not admit patients—pathologists, anesthesiologists, radiologists—are more likely to lose admitting privileges when other physicians of the same specialty win exclusive contracts with their hospital. On the other hand, insurers now readily use claims databases to profile physicians' practice habits before winnowing their networks. Profiling by insurers, if not discriminatory by race, sex, age, or religion (creed), is deemed legal by the courts, because clinicians are considered vendors, not customers, and excluding individual physicians from provider networks does not diminish competition. Insurers may eliminate one-third to one-half of physicians from their older PPOs, preferring more restricted networks of physicians with more "efficient" practice profiles. Profiling by insurers is a much greater economic threat to most physicians than profiling by hospitals.

Hospitals began profiling physicians because of the change by Medicare to prospective payment in 1983, putting hospitals at financial risk for inpatient costs of Medicare patients. However, hospitals have generally been ambivalent about alerting physicians about the profiling they have done in administration, because most physicians also admit patients under 65 years of age, most of whom still have some form of indemnity insurance that pays a hospital more for each day the patient stays in the hospital. Hospitals may invest in profiling software, but they usually do not share the data with clinical departments for fear of antagonizing physicians and losing their admissions. Instead, physicians who seem to use more resources on Medicare patients than the hospital can afford may be advised by administration in a quiet way. They are shown how the financial outcomes of their patients compare to the average for similar patients, usually defined by diagnosis-related group (DRG). Most physicians in most hospitals are not shown how the outcomes of their patients compare to those of other physicians in departmental meetings.

A number of early reports of hospitals' profiling the practice habits of physicians were reviewed in 1993.[1] A 1989 survey of 3,400 hospitals determined that only 5 percent of hospitals then had programs in operation to review physicians' utilization of resources for inpatients and their associated costs. A 1991 survey of 500 hospitals found that 40 percent would consider physicians' economic performance in credentialing; 2 percent indicated they regularly prepared and used physician-specific profiles for educational purposes. A 1993 survey of 55 member hospitals of the University Health Systems Consortium found that 66 percent developed and reviewed profiles of physicians. However, only two-thirds of those that did so (44 percent of the total) shared the profiles with their medical staffs, and only 35 percent of them collected and included economic data elements. As late as 1993, 40 of the 48 academic medical centers indicated their boards of trustees were very remote from issues of physician profiling and economic credentialing.

The number of hospitals and PHOs investing in physician profiling and continuing education for medical staff members based on the results of such profiling will increase as hospital operating margins decline. Few hospitals, even in 1999, are prepared to analyze the clinical and financial outcomes of physicians' practice patterns and to share those data with clinicians. Most PHOs do not have the epidemiological expertise or budgets for health data analysis, practice profiling, and risk adjustment that would allow them to develop practice guidelines for their clinicians. Nor do they have clinical, financial, and functional status data on processes of care and outcomes in an electronic format that would permit rapid practice profiling and outcome analysis. Most hospitals face the daunting task of marshaling resources for retrospective, manual chart review if clinical departments express interest in systematic study of the clinical and financial outcomes of their patients. Clinical departments of most hospitals include competitors who have less incentive to invest their time to help colleagues improve practice habits than they would if they were all in the same economic unit, a group practice. But most group practices do not have suitable data for profiling and have less money for data analysis than do hospitals.

Nevertheless, there has been growing interest in profiling physicians' practice habits among physician groups that are at financial risk. The commercial information systems most hospitals acquire for such profiling use the same basic data set of inpatient claims—the UB-92 data set. The data elements include demographic identifiers of the patient (birth date, sex, race, discharge status); up to nine diagnoses and up to six procedures; and the sum of charges by major type of service, such as pharmacy, laboratory, radiology, physical therapy, dietary, nursing, and operating room. These data are very limited for practice profiling. They do not include outpatient data. There are no findings from physical examinations, no laboratory results, no pharmaceuticals identified by name, and no measures of patients' functional status before or after treatment. Risk adjustment in most of these commercial systems currently depends on age, sex, diagnosis, and procedure codes alone. They explain less than half the variation in outcomes they measure, and the UB-92 only includes three outcomes—length of stay, charges, and discharge statistics.

None of the most popular commercial systems for profiling physicians' practice habits in hospitals explains more than half the variation in charges, length of stay, or mortality rates, the three major outcomes measured by these systems. Much of the variation in outcomes is not explained by the limited data collected for profiling. In the future, these systems will be far less important than those now emerging that adjust for risk and profile physicians' practice habits across the continuum of care.

In the past 10 years, the proportion of U.S. health care expenditures spent in hospitals has declined from 50 percent to less than 40 percent, much less in areas where physicians have strong financial incentives to manage their patients out of hospital. The average number of hospital bed days for a representative population of people under 65 years of age has declined in the past 10 years from more than 700 days per 1,000 people per year to less than 200 in many areas where health maintenance organizations and capitation are prevalent. In regions where competition among health plans for members and among providers for patients is most fierce, far less than half the total per capita funds for health care services are spent in hospitals. Hospitals rarely have data on what happens to patients outside their facilities, unless they self-insure for the health care benefits of their employees and can analyze claims data from their care.

For all these reasons, hospitals have not been, and probably never will be, the center of attention for profiling physicians' performance. The center of attention in health care policy and economics has shifted from the hospital to the health plan and the physician-hospital organization. Funds devoted to physician profiling flow to institutions that collect and analyze data on members (those who use clinical resources and those who do not) and on patients who receive care in many settings, over time.

In the mid-1980s, interest in provider profiling emerged in the employer community. It focused on the outcomes of physicians and hospitals and was led by employer coalitions concerned about rising health care costs and impressed with small area variation studies. Employer coalitions in Cleveland and Cincinnati, Ohio; Rochester, New York; and Los Angeles, California convinced, or coerced, hospitals to fund the collection and analysis of discharge abstract data for public distribution of profiles. Today, several for-profit firms have begun posting hospital and physician profiles on the Internet. Visit www.the healthpages.com for profiles of physicians, and www.healthcarereportcards.com for report cards on hospitals.

In most of the programs, providers do not take the initiative to measure themselves. The providers do not keep the data for analysis; employer coalitions, state agencies, and entrepreneurs do. Most important, the data are not complete enough for the keepers of the data to say why wide variation existed in the costs of health care for apparently similar patients. The

# Physician Profiling

processes for data collection start in motion in board rooms far removed from where care is delivered to patients, and physicians are put in the position of defending the differences, usually by criticizing the methodologies for data collection and analysis. Occasional reminders from some distant evaluative organization that length of stay or cost of care is too high does little to motivate a clinical department of competitors to invest their time and resources in systematic evaluation and modification of the processes of care. Receiving general and dated messages that there exists wide variation in practice styles and costs of care will not induce a clinical department of competitors to invest hundreds of hours in thorough data analysis and consideration of alternative processes to improve clinical care and hospital financial performance. They need to have good data, and the fear of God that, if they don't invest the time to improve their clinical practices, very bad things will happen to them.

In 1994, the senior physician executive of Providence Medical Center (PMC), Seattle, Washington, described in detail successful implementation of a physician profiling program that led to quantifiable benefits that substantially exceeded the costs of the program.[2] In the late 1980s, Seattle hospital managers felt financial pressure from managed care plans and the prospective payment system. PMC administration first presented profiling data to the medical staff at that time, but physicians resented the intrusion into their domain and rejected the process, complaining that the data were not valid because they were based on financial claims data, were not risk-adjusted, included outlier cases that ought to have been excluded from the analysis, were not accompanied by local benchmarks for comparisons, produced no summary scoring or relative ranking of physicians that they could understand easily, and were presented without graphics. The medical staff did not receive any training in risk adjustment, in the methods used for profiling, or in interpretation of the data presented to them. After meeting unexpected resistance and contempt from the medical staff, administration abandoned its attempt to influence medical staff practice habits.

Two years later, the competitive climate in Seattle had grown much less comfortable for clinicians. They felt under siege and were aware that they might lose a substantial proportion of their patients to other providers contracting with managed care plans if their patients' outcomes were not as favorable as those of the other providers. Medical staff leaders in 1991 asked administration to organize an outcomes assessment and practice profiling program. With the support of medical staff leaders, administration established a profiling methodology and process that avoided the mistakes made two years earlier. The medical staff approved the selection of All-Payer-Defined DRGs (APR-DRGs) as the risk-adjustment methodology for the program. After careful study, 8 percent of patients' records were removed from the study as outliers. The hospital acquired comparable data on patients from all other state hospitals from the state discharge abstract database.

Every member of each clinical specialty department received his or her data compared to all other physicians in the same department and also compared to peer groups in other hospitals. Every physician had several opportunities to attend a 90-minute presentation on profiling in general and on the data and profiling methodology selected by PMC in particular, followed by a more thorough presentation to each clinical department of its own data and of valid ways of interpreting the data. Each physician received a unique number by which all data were reported, so the data were anonymous. The range of variation discovered for most common DRGs was considerable, more than members of the medical staff expected. Individual counseling and follow-up data analysis were offered to any physician who wanted them.

After release of the first physician profiles, interest in development of practice guidelines appeared for the first time among members of the medical staff. Since then, the hospital has released profiling data every six months, more often for physicians who request it. After one year, a retrospective assessment of the program disclosed a surprisingly large decline in average length of stay (from 5.3 to 4.8 days), accounting for an estimated savings of more than 7,700 hospital bed days and an observation that the hospital appeared to health plans to be a more attractive facility with which to contract. No physicians lost admitting privileges as a result of this profiling project. Most physicians expressed interest in having the program continue.

The profiling programs that will have a much larger (and potentially devastating) influence on physicians are those created by health insurance carriers to winnow their networks of participating physicians by factors of 33 to 66 percent. Insurers are profiling physicians' practice habits and selecting physicians whose habits appear most consistent with "cost-effective" practice. Their means of measuring cost-effective practice (they scrupulously avoid any mention of quality of care) may be challenged, but the effects they can have on physicians' practices are indisputable. Some physicians find themselves losing 10 percent or more of their practices immediately after an insurer drops them from its managed care panel of providers. For instance, in 1993, Blue Cross and Blue Shield of the National Capital Area (BCBSNCA, Washington, D.C.) eliminated one-third of participating physicians from its new preferred provider plan. BCBSNCA used Pro/File, a physician profiling system it developed under the direction of Dr. Ron Klar and now sells to other Blue Cross and Blue Shield plans. King County Medical Blue Shield, Seattle, Washington, removed 40 percent of participating physicians from its approved networks of providers using Pro/File.

Pro/File aggregates claims data into a patient-centered database and allows comparisons of physicians' practice habits over time across multiple outpatient and inpatient visits for all the physicians' patients. Pro/File is used to calculate average consumption of resources for each physician, including diagnostic studies and consultations and hospitalizations, for the most common types of patients he or she treats. Then outcomes (defined in terms of resource consumption) are compared to the norm for the physician's specialty, based on the types and numbers of patients treated. The system finds an expected resource consumption for each type of patient, based on practice habits in the entire metropolitan area, and assigns those expected values to each physician's patient population to determine whether expected resource consumption is higher or lower than actual resource consumption for each physician.[3]

Profiling serves another purpose of managed care firms besides reducing the ranks of contracting physicians. The firms use profiling systems to answer a question posed frequently by employers: "How do you know your doctors are any good?" The only source of information insurers and employers have on the practice habits of physicians is the database of historical claims data insurers maintain for retrospective analysis and profiling of physicians. Insurers with indemnity health insurance business use the claims databases built by those indemnity claims to profile community physicians before they select a subset of them for new managed care plans.

Using claims data presents many challenges to insurers, the largest of which involve reliably identifying patients and providers and tracking all claims filed by or for patients over time to identify resources consumed and ailments treated during an episode of illness.

# Physician Profiling

Physicians complete claims more accurately than ever before, and insurers process them with more edits for reliability than ever before, but claims still too often cannot be linked reliably to the appropriate physicians or patients. Physicians are suspicious of any evaluation of their practice habits based on claims data, because they know claims are often completed haphazardly and may include only one diagnosis code when a variety of services were rendered.

Recognizing these limitations, insurers have still moved ahead to profile physicians using claims data, knowing that the data are more reliable in tightly managed health plans that assign patients to primary physicians and penalize them financially for obtaining services out of network. Insurers profile primary care physicians by calculating expected patterns of outpatient resource consumption by common types of patients (sometimes stratified into gender and age categories) and by deriving a separate model for each type of primary care physician (pediatrician, family physician, and general internist). Once expected patterns of resource consumption are developed for each specialty for common types of patients, usually defined by common ailments, each physician's results are compared to expectations. Because most insurers cannot be confident that they can track all the services rendered to patients over time, or which physician is responsible for which services, profiling is done by visit, comparing physicians' use of resources by type of visit for type of patient. Physicians are compared on the basis of their relative total outpatient charges per type of office visit, per diagnosis code, per period (when all claims are submitted to the insurer for any given patient). Other comparisons include relative need for follow-up appointments and additional treatments within 90 days of the first office visit, relative use of consultations during a defined treatment process, relative use of laboratory and radiology services, relative number of visits per person per year, and relative level of intensity of services provided in office visits.

The use of the word relative calls attention to the need for some kind of risk adjustment. There are two general types of risk adjustment for outpatient services—visit-based and person-based. When the insurer is confident that all claims for services to individual patients are filed and that it has a complete database of claims for specific populations of patients, person-based risk adjustment, also called population-based risk adjustment, leads to more accurate adjustment for risk. The three best known systems for population-based risk adjustment are Ambulatory Care Groups (ACGs) from Johns Hopkins University, Peer-A-Med from HealthChex, and Episode Treatment Groups. When payers do not have all the claims for individuals, they use visit-based risk adjustment, such as Ambulatory Visit Groups, Products of Ambulatory Care, Ambulatory Severity Index, Products of Ambulatory Surgery, and Ambulatory Patient Groups. The latter system, a methodology developed by 3M Healthcare, has been selected by the Health Care Financing Administration for reimbursement of Medicare outpatient services.

The focus of cost containment and outcomes management has expanded to the entire continuum of care. More and more Americans each month receive their care from health care systems of providers that accept a global capitation for their services for a defined population over a specified period. Those delivery systems want their physicians to understand how they compare to their peers, and they want them to work together to improve the effectiveness and efficiency of their work. The average total costs of care for a physician's panel of patients is a much more important indicator of clinical performance to a capitated delivery system than hospital, outpatient, or consultants costs above.

Insurers and health plans that have access to their own claims data are licensing profiling systems so they can measure and predict the resources needed to care for specific populations of patients. With these models of expected resource consumption, health plans are profiling physicians, comparing their results to those the model would predict, budgeting for staff and resources for ambulatory treatment facilities, and credentialing physicians.

In summary, physicians should expect to be profiled and to receive profiling results from hospitals, group practices, PHOs, and health plans. I suggest that physicians try to get profiled and insist that the organizations in which they work or the systems of care in which they see patients invest in staff and information systems to profile them. Outcome measurement for patients and subsequent profiling of physicians by the outcomes of their patients are the first two steps on the road to continuous quality improvement. Without comparative data, physicians and their organizations will compete for managed care contracts without a clear sense of how competitive they are.

Once your clinical community has selected a methodology for collection and analysis of patient data, a team consisting of clinicians trained in epidemiology and a statistician will prove invaluable in helping clinicians whose care is profiled to understand the methodology used, its weaknesses and strengths, and how to inquire into the data set beyond the initial reports a commercial system may produce. Sharing the data with clinicians in an educational way is key to successful cultural change. Physicians are learners. They want to interrogate data and see how their performance compares to that of their peers. The process needs grounding in valid clinical research methods and in continuing education for professionals.

**References**

1. Riley, D. "Economic Credentialing Survey of University Teaching Hospitals." *Healthcare Financial Management* 47(12):42-54, Dec. 1993.

2. Bennett, G., and others. "Case Study of Physician Profiling." *Managed Care Quarterly* 2(4):60-70, Autumn 1994.

3. Ron Klar, MD, Blue Cross and Blue Shield of the National Capital Area, personal communication.

# Chapter 26
## Informatics and Practice Guidelines

After profiling, what's next? What comes after you have used claims data to profile the processes and outcomes of care of your health care delivery system? After you have seen the substantial variation that exists between clinicians in their ways of managing patients, what do you do? Do you send out a notice to all clinicians that substantial variation exists? Do you produce individual report cards and mail them to clinicians? Do you organize continuing education programs to teach new practice habits? Do you sigh in dismay and long for those relatively uncontroversial morbidity and mortality meetings? Do you organize chart review sessions for clinicians with the worst process and outcome measures? Do you ignore the indicators because practice variation identified in claims data does not warrant closer scrutiny or because physicians vary dramatically in the ways in which they select diagnosis and procedure codes and complete claims? Do you ignore variation because you find the process and outcome indicators of most clinicians still fall within two standard deviations of the mean? Realize that, even with large-scale variation in outcome indicators of patients, 95 percent of clinicians will produce results within two standard deviations of the mean. That's the way the normal distribution works. No matter how much variation exists among those physicians, if their results are distributed normally, 95 percent of them will have results that fall within the normal range.

Imagine that the variation among family physicians in their referral rates to subspecialists is such that a 40-fold difference exists between the lowest and the highest referral rate to any given specialty. One physician is 40 times more likely than another to refer his or her patients to any particular subspecialist. In a normal distribution of physicians' referral rates, a 30- or 35-fold difference might not be statistically significant as long as a few other physicians differ in their referral rates by more. So, what do you do? Do you set your confidence limits at one standard deviation from the mean referral rate, and so identify roughly one-third of the physicians as outliers with "abnormal" referral rates? Or do you take the other extreme and set your normal range at three standard deviations from the mean, and only identify one physician in a thousand whose referral rate falls outside of three standard deviations from the mean? Or do you do nothing?

Because the statistical definition of abnormal that we use in medicine (those observations falling outside of two standard deviations away from the mean) identifies so few physicians as "abnormal" (only 5 percent, to be precise), identifying them may not be worth your while. Next month, a different set of physicians will have results outside two standard deviations from the mean, and the ones abnormal last month may be normal the next month.

If you do nothing, do you rationalize your inactivity by noting that insurers don't want to limit their provider networks anyway, even if it means eliminating clinicians whose care is substandard? Do you decide you cannot act on a clinician with certain indicators more than two standard deviations from the mean because the risk-adjustment method only explains about half the variation in the outcome selected for risk adjustment? What do you do when a clinician's report card is poor in one area but excellent in another? What do you do when he or she uses radiology services very sparingly, but refers to certain subspecialists or prescribes pharmaceuticals far more often than expected?

Not only does substantial variation in the practices of clinicians occur in most organized delivery systems, but the statistical methods for evaluating care retrospectively often do not have enough precision to help medical directors distinguish results due to random variation among patients from results due to the variable practice habits of clinicians. Add to this mix the variation introduced by administrative staff who complete the billing records (claim forms) that produce the data used by most profiling systems of payers and providers. Substantial variation in the observed process and outcome indicators may be due to variation introduced by billing habits of administrative staff. Is the office practice with claims showing large numbers of complicated patients burdened with sicker patients or up-coding routine office visits to maximize reimbursement? Most clinicians will assume the patients are more challenging or demanding. Most insurers will assume the office maximizes reimbursement with aggressive coding practices. Physicians are usually surprised at the cynical perspective insurers take to evaluation of clinicians' billing practices. Physicians suffer from the burdensome reporting requirements of distrusting insurers. Insurers suffer from the aggressive, some would say fraudulent, billing practices of some medical groups.

When you study variation in health care results, you quickly notice that substantial variation exists. After you study the causes of variability, you may not, with confidence, be able to distinguish appropriate from inappropriate care. You will look for patterns that recur over time, of the physician or medical group that routinely orders the most tests, the most consultations, the most surgical procedures or that has the least appealing outcomes of care. If you use the 95 percent confidence intervals of two standard deviations from the mean as your arbitrary dividing line between observations that could have, and could not have, occurred by random variation alone, you will only identify 5 percent of the physicians or medical groups as outliers at any particular point in time, even if some of them differ from others by 20-fold, 30-fold, even 40-fold in rates of process and outcome measures.

So, you may abandon the goal of identifying normal and abnormal practices by process and outcome indicators all together and publish process and outcome indicators in report cards for all to see. You may enlist the assistance of clinical leaders to design practice guidelines that you will ask clinicians to learn and follow whenever they can to reduce observed variation in care.

## After Profiling Come Guidelines

After data analysis and distribution of indicator sets in the form of report cards come visits to outlying physicians by various physicians and nurses involved in quality assurance and utilization management. But in order to change everyone's practice habits and reduce variation in processes and outcomes in the health care system, you will have to define expected practices and teach them to clinicians. We can teach expected practice habits by establishing guidelines for care and by making them available and familiar to clinicians. Clinicians learn medical care by guidelines. Medical students study guidelines in lecture notes from the medical faculty. Nurses learn guidelines in nursing school. Residents learn to find guidelines in textbooks and handbooks of medical practice. Guidelines appear everywhere in medical education. If the patient has certain symptoms, physical findings, and laboratory results, treat him this way, with this regimen. On the other hand, if he presents with these findings, treat him that way. The exercise of prescribing a treatment is an effort to assign a guideline for care to an individual patient with a specific set of characteristics. A guideline lists the services expected for patients with specific characteristics.

Guidelines do not represent mandatory care. They suggest expected care, unless extenuating circumstances (that occur all too often) warrant deviation from the guideline. Screening guidelines will apply to a majority of people in the age and sex cohorts to which they apply. Treatment guidelines may apply to only a minority of people with a given ailment because of extenuating circumstances. Some patients whom guidelines will say should take a certain medication do not receive that medication because they have developed an allergic reaction to it. Treatment guidelines often need modification because of allergies, comorbid conditions, other medications, or recent medical history. The patient who has had bilateral total mastectomies does not need a screening mammogram. The patient with a personal history of colonic polyps needs screening for colon cancer by colonoscopy more often than members of the general public do.

## Guidelines Are a Natural Extension of Management Control

In a management control system, there are (1) inputs, (2) a conversion process, (3) outputs, and, for management control, (4) sensors, (5) standards of production that determine the measurements of the sensors, and (6) a control process that acts on the inputs or conversion process when the sensor indicates the output of the process is not consistent with the goals set for the process.[1] For management control of a health care process to succeed, the sensors need to monitor production of services such as quality of care, resources consumed, patient satisfaction, and functional status.

If the process and outcome measures of the conversion process are not acceptable, clinical management control needs to intervene. The corrective action taken could involve education and training of the clinicians involved in the process to the state of the art in medical care (usually defined as a guideline or set of related guidelines). Corrective action could include procedural change in the way clinicians are asked to practice or a change in the personnel who carry out the conversion process. Perhaps the poor outcomes involve patients who have not prepared for a conversion process (arriving for a colonoscopy without having prepped their bowels) and who need different instructions and incentives to prepare successfully for certain procedures. Then, again, perhaps the clinicians or the patients need incentives, or disciplinary action, to motivate them to follow the rules of the conversion process. Finally, some patients, and some clinicians, who fail to follow the rules of a practice need to be removed from the managed care plan.

Management control systems depend on standards for inputs, conversion processes, and outcomes of a process. Without established standards, we cannot define our expectations for a process or the results of the process. A clinical practice guideline codifies our expectations for inputs, the features of treatment, and the outcomes that represent the output of the process. With an established practice guideline and a modern information system to identify inputs, conversion process steps, and outcomes of care, we can automate some of the surveillance that goes with the goal of delivering state-of-the-art care and of continuously improving care. Think of clinical practice guidelines as formalized expectations used to guide clinicians to deliver optimal care. Clinical practice guidelines determine what information is stored in the information systems used to automate record keeping and monitoring of care.

## When Will Practice Guidelines Be Put into Computers?

At the moment, most health care institutions have simple clinical protocols printed on paper for most clinicians to memorize and recall when they see a patient for whom a particular protocol applies. In a setting with many protocols, such as in a cancer center with numerous clinical research protocols under evaluation simultaneously, one can find a protocol book that has the protocols and their steps printed. Patients on a specific protocol will often have one or more flow sheets in their charts telling clinicians what steps have been accomplished and which have yet to be performed. In most settings, the protocols are in analog (paper) form. In the few settings in which the protocols can be retrieved electronically, they resemble static electronic documents viewed on a screen instead of on paper. It is the rare clinical setting today where you will find an automated, digital medical record that electronically reports a patient's status with respect to a protocol as the patient receives care.

You will not find digital medical records in which clinicians enter their findings about patients in a structured database stored in a computer except in a few clinics in a few academic medical centers intentionally studying the benefits and costs of computer-based patient records. There are more medical records in electronic form, but most are created by storing clinicians' transcribed dictation and cannot be searched reliably by computers to ascertain which patients are, and which are not, receiving care according to established protocols. Free text dictation does not lend itself to reliable digital analysis by computer because clinicians have so many ways of expressing the same concept and so many ways of ordering their findings that we cannot effectively and efficiently parse what clinicians dictate into standardized, structured databases. Consequently, the clinical guidelines that are automated are fairly rudimentary. There is a guideline to which most clinicians would ascribe without reservation that stipulates not to prescribe for patients medications to which they have had known allergic reactions. A computer can store a patient's allergies in digital form and check that drugs ordered for that patient do not have known allergic potential for that patient. Companies such as First Data and Multum and PHAMIS (IDX) market products that check tables of allergies for potential adverse drug reactions before processing orders for pharmaceuticals.

Because data about patients are not in structured databases, most clinicians do not have access to automated systems that search for potential drug or allergic reactions or for patients whose care is not following established protocols. We will not see computer systems that suggest protocols for patients until we have computers that store detailed data about patients—demographics, history, physical examination, laboratory results, and pharmacy data—in structured databases that rules-based logic can work on automatically. At the moment, the digital nurse may enter physicians' orders into a computer and the digital physician may retrieve laboratory results from a computer, but computers are not—in all but a few experimental settings—giving clinicians advice about how to treat patients. They do not have data on patients in structured, standardized electronic format on which their logic can work. The political and social costs of collecting standardized structured data in electronic form are simply too high.

## Impediments to Collecting Structured Data

Most physicians are not paid by the hour. Physicians paid under fee-for-service arrangements earn a living by piecework—the more services they render, the more income they earn. Managed care contracts have reduced the income to most physicians by paying less for services than they once received from insurers. Medicare instituted relative value units to pay for procedures and reduced the pay to many procedural physicians considerably. Physicians feel they must see more patients and perform more procedures just to keep up with inflation and pay their bills. Physicians paid capitation earn more money the more health plan members are assigned to their care. The more members under capitation, the more patients in the waiting room, on the telephone, and in the hospital that they must evaluate and treat. So, either under capitation or under fee for service, physicians feel compelled to minimize the time spent with patients, to see as many patients as possible in a give period. Physicians do not earn more money for taking the time to collect structured, standardized data about their patients.

In this setting, any new procedure for keeping records that slows a physician down during his or her daily work will be rejected. Most computer-based patient records with structured databases depend on physicians to perform the data entry, using a mouse and a keyboard to select data from menus to describe a patient. Few physicians find a mouse and a keyboard a more efficient way to collect data about patients than the pen and paper or dictating equipment.

It is true that, in most hospitals, computers contain and communicate demographic information, laboratory results, pharmaceuticals, and orders in electronic form. Most group practices do not have those data in electronic form, but, with maturation of office practice systems, more will have them. The problem for automation of clinical practice guidelines is that the data from physicians' histories and physicals are not automated in structured electronic form. While computers give piecemeal advice about drug-drug interactions, most physicians do not enter their own orders to benefit from advice presented on a computer screen. Because computers do not store in structured, electronic form the histories and the physical examinations of most patients, or their physicians' assessments of them, most of the information that would establish suitable clinical protocols for those patients is not available to computers to act on. And physicians are not likely to take the time to type or click in all the data needed for a computer to give back a useful judgment about whether or not a patient's specific circumstances warrant a specific clinical practice guideline.

There are exceptions to the general rule of physicians' antipathy to electronic medical records. House officers and fellows in medical centers are paid to collect information about patients and may be expected to complete electronic medical records. Not long ago, the Medical Center of the University of Virginia (UVA) learned that even usually docile house officers have a threshold for inconvenience and inefficiency in record keeping beyond which they will not voluntarily venture. The UVA house staff initially refused to work with an electronic medical record system thrust upon them by hospital administration. The system was implemented anyway, and the house staff generally regards it with approval. On the other hand, a majority of office practices in England and Norway use electronic medical records for patients, although the data are not structured in a precise or standardized way. Physicians at the Medical Center of Indiana University and at the affiliated Regenstrief Institute in Indianapolis have used the Regenstrief Medical Record for more than 10 years to keep structured electronic records about patients. The Regenstrief system has included automated guidelines for years, with published research confirming the value of automated alerts and reminders to house physicians about when patients need services according to guidelines established in the medical center.

Tradition does play a substantial role in physicians' acceptance of electronic medical records. Physicians applying for privileges to practice at institutions using electronic records know they will use electronic records. In this circumstance, physicians' resistance to electronic medical records is muted. In institutions where physicians must abandon old habits of paper records or transcription to learn data entry with a keyboard and mouse, resistance may be fierce, unless the physicians believe an electronic record will save them time and money.

**Creating Guidelines Is a Labor of Love**
Guidelines must be implemented to be useful. Most of our efforts in creating guidelines have been for development, and relatively little, much too little, effort has been invested in implementing guidelines. A set of guidelines of hundreds of pages each of inextricable branching logic, as some of the PORT studies of the Agency for Health Care Policy and Research (AHCPR) produced, will not be adopted and followed by physicians. Physicians will not take the time to sort through multiple pages of logic and algorithms to find the appropriate guideline for a given patient. Instead, they will rely on their memories and best judgment, and all too often produce idiosyncratic practice habits unique to each individual clinician. Guidelines must be simple enough for clinicians to remember and be made available to physicians while they see patients to remind them of the process steps that patients who fit the guideline are expected to follow. Before adoption and implementation, guidelines should be studied, and probably modified by physicians expected to follow them to meet the exigencies of local facilities and available staff. Successful implementation of a guideline requires incentives (positive or negative reinforcement), awareness, constant reminders, and systematic profiling of those who do, and do not, follow the guideline that has been adopted by their clinical community.

Information systems can play a valuable role in supporting implementation of clinical practice guidelines in several ways. Theoretically, a computer can obtain all relevant information about a patient and use Bayesian logic to formulate a guideline suitable for that patient's specific circumstances. But, notice the word, "theoretically." In practice, we are decades from all but the simplest feedback loops in computers that give clinicians guidance in managing patients in the office or hospital. The primary impediment to application of rules-based logic in computers to give advice to clinicians is data collection. Computers require data in digital form. Someone has to enter the data about patients and treatments into digital form. While data entry has grown much more efficient with the advent of bar code readers, automatic analyzers, light pens, mice and keyboards, even speech recognition, the detailed findings of clinicians still reside impregnable in the paper record. However, with the advent of predictive modeling of outcomes and automation of practice guidelines, we will see serious investment in training and technology for electronic records in order to collect data and calculate the expected outcomes that will help clinicians follow specific clinical guidelines for specific

# *Informatics and Practice Guidelines*

patients at specific points in time. In 50 years, those electronic records and automated clinical guidelines will be as indispensable to physicians as the stethoscope became to physicians after its technology improved and they overcame their opposition to removing their ears from patients' chests.

## References

1. Austin, C., and Boxerman, S. *Information Systems for Health Services Administration,* Fifth Edition. Chicago, Ill.: Health Administration Press, 1997, p. 32.

# Chapter 27

# The Importance of Data Warehouses for Physician Executives

Soon, most physicians will begin to learn about data warehouses and about clinical and financial data about their patients stored in them. What is a data warehouse? Why are we seeing their emergence in health care now? How does a hospital, group practice, PHO, or health plan acquire or create a data warehouse? Who should be responsible for it, and what sort of training is needed by those in charge of using it?

Physicians are just beginning to learn that insurers have been building data warehouses of claims data for years and use those databases to determine which physicians and provider organizations to contract with in new, more "selective" preferred provider networks. When a physician is excluded from a managed care contract because the insurer has decided that he or she has shown "uneconomical" practice patterns in the past, as determined by analysis of a claims database, the physician has little recourse without access to a data warehouse that shows his or her practice is in the mainstream of medical care. The vast majority of physicians and hospitals have no such data warehouses at their disposal. Some PHOs are developing them to help their affiliated physicians study outcomes of care and identify processes of care that can be improved.

A data warehouse for health care populations consists of integrated information about patients, their symptoms and signs of disease, their diagnoses and procedures, their clinical laboratory and radiology results, and their charges and associated costs in a relational database useful for clinical and health services research studies. Data warehouses contain millions of records about hundreds of thousands, in some cases millions, of patients. The data warehouses of insurance companies have claims data from HCFA1500 and UB92 claims filed with procedures, diagnoses, charges, and payments. Insurers usually do not have access to clinical data, such as laboratory and radiology reports, so those important details will not be in the data warehouses they build. Conversely, data warehouses that providers build will have inpatient and outpatient claims data, laboratory and radiology results, and pharmaceutical data, but they will not include data about patients treated by competitors. If providers have cost accounting systems, they may include in their data warehouse data on charges, payments, and costs associated with services.

To the best of my knowledge, no large group practice, hospital, or health care system has an enterprise data warehouse with clinical and financial details of care plus standardized measures of the functional status of patients, both before and after treatment. Standards for identifying diagnoses (ICD-9-CM) and procedures (ICD-9-CM and CPT4) are fairly well developed and are widely used by providers, because most providers in the civilian health care system are paid for their services on a piece-rate, fee-for-service basis that requires identification of diagnoses and procedures for payment. But there are no widely used standards for defining patients' symptoms or physicians' findings on physical examinations of patients. They have not needed to identify symptoms or findings for reimbursement. Why do they need to collect those data now? Because buyers of health care services are beginning to ask sellers of health care insurance, either managed care plans or provider organizations directly contracting with employers, to produce evidence of acceptable clinical outcomes and to show continuous improvement in those outcomes.

In the past, group- and staff-model health maintenance organizations shadow-priced indemnity insurance health plans, pricing their insurance products about 10 percent below the high-option indemnity plans and still offering more generous services. Staff- and group-model HMOs, such as Kaiser Permanente Health Plan, never needed to collect detailed HCFA 1500 forms for the office visits of their patients, because they did not produce bills for service. Now, as competing integrated health care delivery systems begin to emerge in the previously fragmented, private practice community of providers, even Kaiser needs systematic and standardized data collection for all the services rendered to all its members. Kaiser needs to create a database its leaders can use to analyze patterns of treatment, institute systematic quality improvement, and compete for patients more effectively. So does the military health system, which finds itself in need of data analysis and reporting systems to help its leaders compare their health care system to the civilian systems with which they compete for Tricare beneficiaries.

Where should the data be stored that physicians and hospitals collect electronically for patient care and billing, data that they want to study to identify opportunities to reduce costs and improve quality of patient care? The data should flow into an electronic data warehouse. Physician-hospital organizations (PHOs) will achieve a significant competitive advantage over disorganized providers and health plans once they pool their clinical and administrative data into data warehouses for systematic study.

All too often, data in electronic form are printed on paper to produce bills and laboratory and pharmacy reports and then are purged from electronic storage after patients have completed office visits or have been discharged from hospital. Chief financial officers may be delighted to print data on paper, because they think paper storage of medical and administrative records is cheaper than electronic storage on magnetic disk drives, optical disk drives, or magnetic tape. Because they have never suffered through chart review, however, CFOs do not understand the hideous inefficiency of abstracting clinical data from paper records in order to perform clinical research, quality improvement, and utilization and risk management studies.

Computer technologies are becoming more robust, less expensive, and more efficient faster than the attitudes of most health care managers are changing about those technologies. The principal assets of a health care organization are its medical records. Organizations need to realize that continuous quality improvement requires frequent, ad hoc access to data about the processes that may need improvement. Organizations can facilitate quality improvement studies and reduce the expensive hours spent in manual data collection by investing once in the creation of a corporate data warehouse that will serve many users countless times in their searches for data.

Intermountain Health Care discovered that an adequate study of a well-defined clinical process still required some $50,000 in time by medical record specialists abstracting several hundred clinical details from 1,000 charts. Why so many charts? There are so many variations in the conditions of patients before a surgical procedure or a medical treatment, so many variations in treatment, and so many ways that patients may respond to treatments that large numbers of patients need to be studied to identify statistically significant trends attributable to treatment. It makes far more sense to copy clinical and financial data from transaction systems to a data warehouse than to grope through paper records containing data that were at one time in electronic form in transaction systems.

Physicians readily embrace the concept of a data warehouse for health services and clinical research on their own patient populations. Physicians have not been given clinical data about the outcomes of their patients compared to the outcomes of similar patients treated by other physicians in their communities. Physicians are trained in academic health centers where clinical research studies occur every day. They are familiar with standardized data collection and data analysis. Given reliable data about patient outcomes, they will change practice habits and adopt practice guidelines that lead to improvement in the outcomes of care for their patients.

Until a health care organization invests in a data warehouse for integration of clinical, financial, and outcomes data, claims of commitment to quality improvement made by administration ought not to be taken seriously. No organization benefits from managers (and clinicians) squandering countless hours in committee meetings about quality improvement trying to imagine root causes of problems, when they could be analyzing large clinical databases to find important relationships between process and outcome indicators.

The data warehouse is a gold mine in which to find opportunities for clinical quality improvement. Leaders of an organization who choose not to build a data warehouse are saying they are not interested in putting sources of data in the hands of users at an economical price for quality improvement activities. They are more interested in the appearances of quality improvement, which they control, than in widespread pursuit of CQI studies, which cannot be in their control. This resource is too valuable to be left in the hands of managers who may be threatened by the undermining of organizational hierarchy that widespread access to corporate data about patients can produce. Physician managers, who have an understanding of both organizational and clinical needs, are in the best position to champion the creation of data warehouses in their organizations.

# Chapter 28

# Telemedicine: Where Is Technology Taking Us?

About 1990, a few zealots in Switzerland, at the CERN Laboratory, contemplated using the Internet for hypertext and for transfer of still images, recorded sounds, and compressed video files. Today, the World Wide Web defines a set of standards for packaging and routing information over the Internet that involves millions of people and personal computers and that allowed a start-up Netscape to enjoy a capitalization of more than $2 billion when it sold stock to the public. About 1995, videoconferencing and multimedia electronic mail over the Internet fascinated the engineers at NASA; today they are mainstream applications for the Web. Five years from now, you may be participating in telemedicine sessions frequently, from your workstation, over the Internet and think nothing of it.

Most telemedicine trials involve expensive (more than $50,000 per site) and bulky videoconferencing equipment. These devices give physicians the opportunity to see patients on large screens. In these situations, the consultant and the primary physician, with the patient, interact via videoconference in a "live" session. But the expense of the equipment precludes many sites for consultation.

Another hindrance to greater use of telemedicine is the difficulty of scheduling two busy clinicians to confer by videoconference. By their nature, the "live" sessions using television technologies require major investment in production equipment and substantial time devoted by both patients and physicians. While a telemedicine session may save a patient valuable time he or she would otherwise have to spend driving hundreds of miles to a distant referral center, it is unlikely that live television-style videoconferences will be the dominant form of telemedicine because of the expense of equipment and the inconvenience of scheduling a live session for two physicians, one at each location.

In most situations in which a physician wants counsel from another physician on the best way to manage a patient, each physician can benefit substantially from an asynchronous consultation. The physician requesting a consultation can take textual (clinical chemistry) and graphic (ECG) laboratory results and still (x-rays, images from endoscopes) and moving (cardiac catheterization cineangiography) images, store them in digital format, and transport them electronically over communication lines to reside in a multimedia consultation "folder"—a form of multimedia electronic mail—on the workstation of the consultant. After the consultant has studied the folder, he or she will call the physician requesting the consultation to review his or her interpretation of the data and make a recommendation. This is much faster and less expensive than overnight delivery of physical documents and does not require the primary and consulting physicians to be present at a live television session. This is an asynchronous telemedicine consultation and will grow in favor as bandwidth increases and physicians work within capitated health care delivery systems.

NASA has always been a leading user of the Internet. As the digital bandwidth (throughput of data per second) of the Internet increases, NASA and other government agencies are testing the feasibility of videoconferencing over the Internet using the MBONE Information Web that is a subset of the Internet for videoconferencing, just as the World Wide Web is a subset of the Internet for hypertext and graphics. MBONE stands for Multicast Backbone. Live videoconferences take place on the MBONE, using UNIX workstations to receive the multimedia bit streams and to present audio and video components on high-resolution monitors. Today, however, personal computers with Pentium II processors and Windows 98, Windows NT, or OS/2 operating systems have the same capabilities at less cost than the less common UNIX workstations from Silicon Graphics and SUN Microsystems.

Here's the likely scenario for telemedicine to flourish. You are a physician concerned about how to diagnose or treat a particular patient. You have findings from your physical examination of the patient and laboratory studies in digital textual form from a word processor. You have images from one or more diagnostic studies: x-ray, ECG, EEG, and pathology, for example. Those images are also in a computer in digital form, having been scanned, captured by a videocamera, or faxed into digital form. You pull these various forms of information—text, graphics, images, and recorded sounds—on your personal computer into a multimedia electronic mail message, using readily available software from a variety of firms. You send the multimedia document via the Internet to the mailbox of a consultant whose opinion you want for this patient. Your office staff may call the consultant's office to make certain he or she is available to respond to consultation requests today. You set a time, perhaps late in the afternoon, when the consultant can contact you for a conversation to discuss the case, once he or she has had a chance to consider what you have sent. Images and graphics make all the difference. It is difficult to describe over the telephone the x-ray image of a fractured ankle or a pathology slide from a biopsy of a soft tissue tumor. Far better to send a multimedia electronic mail message with the images attached.

You go on about your business, and the consultant calls just before you see your last patient. You want to talk to the consultant, so you tell the patient that you may be on the telephone for 10 minutes, and you go into your office. But you don't just pick up the telephone. Instead you sit in front of your computer and start a videoconference with the consultant, using the MBONE Information Web. You can see the consultant, and he or she can see you, in small windows on your monitors, and you can both see the images and text that you sent in the multimedia message earlier in the day. The consultant has had time to study the information, so your interactive consultation takes less time.

The consultant asks a few questions about your patient concerning information in your transmission that was not clear. You make a mental note to include such data in the future. The consultant uses a mouse to point out on the images you have sent, that you both are looking at on your monitors, those pathognomonic findings that would lead the consultant to treat

## Telemedicine: Where Is Technology Taking Us?

your patient in the way he or she recommends. You listen, take notes, or record the session to transcribe what the consultant says to be part of the medical record for your patient. After a few minutes, you both sign off, and you go back to your last patient of the afternoon. You have practiced telemedicine, but you did it with personal computers and multimedia electronic mail, rather than with expensive television equipment and production personnel.

Now, truth be told, the scenario just described will not happen in a fee-for-service medical economy in which the consultant must bill an insurance company for his contributions to the care of the patient. Insurance companies will not pay for telemedicine consultations. They require consultants to examine patients directly, physically, for payment. They do not know how to regulate telemedicine, which they fear could proliferate uncontrollably if reimbursed. Telemedicine will flourish in capitated systems, in which telemedicine can save money on full consultations avoided and physicians' and patients' time. The current payment system discourages telemedicine, when all other industries are finding ways to use teleconferencing to reduce operating costs and increase the speed of business transactions.

# Chapter 29

## Information Technology: A Way to Streamline Medical Practice

Computers have become indispensable to most businesses for accounting and marketing. Physicians' practices are no exception. As costs increase and revenues decline, information technologies may well be the best investments practices can make for financial, clinical, and marketing reasons. Reduced office expenses, increased revenues, higher patient satisfaction and compliance, and more legible and accessible patient records are among the benefits of implementing information systems. Computer technologies can improve the operations and patient outcomes of office practices. The Internet will become indispensable to link them into a network capable of managing the outcomes and costs of care of defined populations of people over time.

Some physicians swear by computer technology, pointing to reduced office expenses, increased revenue, higher patient satisfaction and compliance, and more legible and accessible patient records. Many managers of firms acquiring physician practices are not interested in investing in office practices that don't have computer technology in place. Malpractice attorneys for the defense implore physicians to use computer technology to make their medical records more legible and complete and to ensure that follow-up appointments are scheduled as needed. They know that computer technology is vital to improving office practice efficiency and patient care.

The electronic patient record depends on networks to access data that are stored on the computers of physicians and provider organizations in various locations. To be truly useful, the records must be shared among providers taking care of populations of people over time, so the data from a visit to an allergist's office are available to the primary physician, as well as to other consultants who might be involved in the patient's care. Not defined by the four walls of a single physician's office, a patient's record achieves its full benefit when the electrons that make it up are available, at the speed of light, at any location within the integrated health care system in which the patient receives care.

There are too many different kinds of office practice systems, and an infinite number of ways of defining the data in them. Physicians' offices need to adopt common data standards, agree on how to define specific fields of data, and share operating systems and application programs. Ideally, physicians should plan their purchase of information systems in concert, so they acquire the hardware, software, and networks and adopt the data standards that allow them to share patient information.

Electronic information exchange between practices depends on networks linking the sites of care. The Internet is becoming that network. Networks (especially the Internet) are more important than the PCs they link, because networks provide access to millions of computers, patients' records, and other valuable information. The PC is a vehicle. You won't get to your destination without roads to lead you there. Those roads are the information super highway, and the Internet is its progenitor.

## Informatics—the New Science

Informatics is a new discipline studying the uses of computer and communication technology to improve information processing. The themes of this science relate to all businesses, all areas of commerce, where people want to use information technology to make their work more effective and efficient. Informatics would not exist as a discipline if we were not in a storm of amazing technological progress in computing and communication technology.

Physicians who want to improve their office practice efficiency and effectiveness and ensure that they will attract payers as well as patients need to learn about informatics. It will help them determine how and where to invest their capital—time and money—in information and communication technology.

## What Makes Informatics Germane to Physicians?

The seminal events in informatics development derive from the discovery at Bell Laboratories, in the late 1940s, of semiconducting materials from which transistors were created in the early 1950s. Transistors can switch the electrical current flowing through them on and off faster, more reliably, and with less power than the vacuum tubes and mechanical relays that were installed in the first computers. Since the discovery of the transistor, manufacturers of electronic devices have learned how to pack more transistors into smaller spaces and how to make them turn on and off at higher speeds, making information processing faster and more reliable.

There were only 6,000 transistors on the 8080 microprocessor from Intel Corporation, the central processing unit for the first personal computer, the Altair, which came in a kit in 1975 and had to be assembled. It was for that personal computer kit that Bill Gates compiled the BASIC programming language and left Harvard to start Microsoft with Paul Allen. Today, there are more than 8,000,000 transistors on the Pentium II microprocessor from Intel. If the 8080 had a data processing power of 1, the data processing power of the Pentium II is more than 2,500 times greater. And the price of the Pentium II is much less than its progenitor chips.

The price of the Pentium II processor is less than that of the 8080 in nominal dollars, and far less in real dollars, adjusted for inflation. In 1974, the 8080 was capable of 0.64 million instructions per second, at a price of $800. In 1998, the Pentium II is capable of 400 million instructions per second, and costs less than $800. The price per million instructions per second has declined from more than $1,250 to less than $1.00.

Electronic memory costs have declined in price and improved in performance just as dramatically. In 1984, the price of 16,000 bytes of electronic memory was $15 per 1,000 bytes storage. In 1998, the price is less than one cent. One byte can store one character—a letter, number, mathematical symbol, or punctuation mark. The cost for permanent memory storage on magnetic hard disk drives has fallen from $220 per megabyte (million bytes) in 1984 to less than 5 cents per megabyte ($240 for 4,800-MB drive) in 1998.

While prices have been falling, the quality of memory storage has increased rapidly, enhancing the added value to consumers even more than these price declines suggest. In 1984, a 1,200-baud (bits per second) modem cost $450, or 38 cents per bit per second. In 1998, an ISDN connector costs $99 for 128,000 bits per second, or .08 cents.

The most dramatic improvements in productivity have come in communicating a bit of information over a telecommunication network: The price has declined substantially. In fact, many people are talking about a foreseeable future in which communicating images, video, voice, and textual data will cost nearly nothing, and the distance those bits of data travel will not materially affect the cost of sending them.

The cost of the hardware (modem) needed to send data over the telephone network in 1984 was about 40 cents per bit per second. The cost of hardware (interface card) needed to send data over a local area network today is .0000099 cents per bit per second. Modems will disappear over the next 10 years as people bring digital telephone and cable TV service into their homes and offices to communicate as fast as, or faster than, they can move data files over local area networks now.

With these dramatic declines in communication costs comes a new phenomenon: The Internet is easily as important to our future as the personal computer was 20 years ago. With the Internet, your computer is connected to millions of other computers all over the world—by local area network, digital telephone, modem, satellite, or cable television. Your PC becomes a window to an electronic universe.

In the 1960s, clerical workers would share one mainframe computer, entering basic accounting information for businesses. In the 1970s, smaller minicomputers designed like small mainframes became available. In health care, department information systems emerged (laboratory, radiology, and pharmacy systems) using those minicomputers. By the 1980s, personal computers appeared, as well as the need to connect them to the corporate computers where much of a company's data were stored.

Large group practices automated their basic accounting and scheduling functions in the late 1970s and 1980s, while small group practices began to automate their administrative records in the late 1980s. Most group practices with more than two physicians have computer systems for business processing. Some early adopters of technology have discovered the benefits of maintaining medical records in electronic form in windowing operating systems, such as Apple Macintosh, Microsoft Windows, or UNIX X-Windows.

Now the stage is set for the next wave of automation in physicians' offices, when they link the information systems of many group practices and hospitals into an electronic web or extranet ("extended Intranet) based on Internet technology. Extranets allow them to move multimedia data about the patients they are treating at the speed of light, to manage the costs of their care as efficiently and effectively as possible.

In the future, the practice that grows in value will be linked electronically to other physicians' offices, share common databases on patients, and participate in the systematic analysis of patient outcomes to reduce costs and enhance care. Success will depend as much on the practice's network as on its internal operations. The network will become an extension of the political network, defined by the managed care organizations with which the practice stakes its future.

## Electronic Information Systems Can Help Your Office Practice

Computerized practice management applications help offices in many ways. Claims tracking is much easier: Users can check on a patient's status with insurers in seconds, and lost or misplaced claims are less likely. Many insurers demand that providers send claims electronically, using software to clean them up before submission. Payers save considerable money by avoiding the cost of entering data on paper claims into their processing systems, and they entice providers to submit electronic claims by paying bonuses to those who do or by reimbursing them promptly.

Ready access to patient information at workstations in the office, via modem at home, and from anywhere else where a computer with compatible client software is attached to a modem gives the electronic record an advantage over the paper variety that is in one place at a time. Physicians can search electronic records in seconds to identify patients for follow-up care and others who need to be notified of a drug recall or a new screening procedure.

Electronic records also lead to more legible and more complete records, because they can alert clinicians when certain data need to be included, which vary with the patient history, clinical findings, and treatments. Electronic records require far less space than that required for analog medical records. The textual contents of 100,000 patients' medical records can be stored on one magnetic hard disk drive costing less than $500 and no larger than a match box. Textual hospital records, minus images, could fit on a disk drive just twice the size, and all images could fit on an optical drive array not much larger than a toaster. Retrieving data on any one patient and searching data of all those patients would be faster because electronic records by design are well-organized and standardized.

Electronic records are important to managed care firms for several reasons, in addition to the efficiencies of electronic claims submission. Utilization management procedures are more often followed, because the electronic records alert clinicians about requirements of health plans for prior approval of certain procedures and treatments. They also provide assistance to clinicians in completing referral forms and preadmission certification for specific payers.

Electronic records include invaluable clinical details for physicians trying to decide whether or not to acquire equipment or add specific clinicians. The database that contains the medical record also includes information about procedures, laboratory studies, and diagnoses that a practice or a hospital can review to identify and count specific patients who might benefit from a new diagnostic or therapeutic device, or from the skills of a subspecialist. They also alert the practice to remind patients of routine and follow-up office visits. Cost-benefit analyses of investments are easier to make with such detailed patient data. Time management can be improved dramatically with electronic records, because they can be used to schedule patients, clinicians, and equipment.

Laboratory results in electronic records can be graphed and trended over time, revealing significant variation in the data that might not be obvious in a tabular listing. Many electronic records that include pharmaceutical and laboratory data allow clinicians to graph variation in physiological parameters, such as white blood cell count, serum creatinine, and SED rate with changing doses of medications.

Electronic medical records usually have features to allow them to print standard reports, including instructions to patients based on diagnoses, procedures, and medications. They also produce standard consultation requests, allowing physicians to copy patients data, attach their comments, and send the data by e-mail to consultants.

Electronic records can give advice to clinicians. Some applications include modules to give advice to patients receiving medications. EMR automatically checks for allergies to prescribed medications, for any contraindications associated with medications, and for the patient's history or physiological parameters, such as renal and hepatic function. Many electronic medical records also will print standardized satisfaction and functional status forms for patients to complete at the appropriate times before and after treatment.

Medical record systems in hospitals and office practices will begin to include images—x-rays, CT and MRI scans, echocardiograms, and ultrasound studies—along with text. Most modern electronic records designed for networks of personal computers and minicomputers accept images already. In the next five years, radiology departments will become totally digital and will produce film only at the request of clinicians. Digital images will be interpreted by radiologists at high-resolution monitors and will be sent to primary care and referring physicians' offices by electronic networks, to be stored on small optical or magnetic disk drives of large capacity.

# Chapter 30

# Information Technology: Interactive Media Enhances Medicine

When all is said and done, we will look back on the late 1990s as the time when we reached a critical mass of computers sharing multimedia information, using the Internet's World Wide Web standards. The shift from personal computing to personal networking is occurring right now. The personal computer has changed from a device primarily for independent computing for authoring documents, to one that gives users access to information on countless other computers around the globe.

Information technology offers physicians myriad options for education, research, and communication. Listed here are some of the interactive media applications that physicians can use to enhance diagnosis, learning, and information sharing.

## Diagnostic Decision Support Systems

Many physicians, primarily internists, are testing diagnostic decision support systems from a variety of developers. These products for personal computers, running under Windows or Macintosh operating systems, originated in academic medical centers for use by house officers and medical students as research projects on mainframe and large minicomputers more than 10 years ago. Quick Medical Reference (QMR) is derived from Internist, developed at the University of Pittsburgh. Iliad was developed at the University of Utah. DXPLAIN was created at Massachusetts General Hospital.

These decision support systems perform like automated textbooks and electronic consultants: Enter a patient's history, including symptoms, findings on physical examination, and diagnostic test results, and the programs will give you a differential diagnosis. The problem for the user is that complex patients with numerous symptoms can require 5 to 15 minutes of data entry. Most physicians will not take so much time during busy clinical work. They may refer to these programs in the evening, at lunch, or on the weekends when they have more time. These programs are expensive for their developers to maintain, because treatments and diagnostic tests change frequently. While these programs tend to serve clinicians well when a patient has one ailment, they often give unrealistic differential diagnoses for patients with more than one simultaneous clinical disorder.

## Therapeutic Decision Support Systems

Therapeutic decision support systems focus on selection and prescription of medications. They automatically check for drug-drug interactions with other prescribed and over-the-counter medications. More sophisticated systems suggest optimal dose and route of administration based on data about the patient's weight, height, age, sex, and organ function. Such systems have been developed for office practices and run on personal computers. The most popular is AskRx Plus from First Data Corporation.

Multum Corporation is creating a sophisticated system for hospital electronic medical records that will advise physicians on medication, dosage, and route of administration based on laboratory findings (creatinine, electrolytes, hemoglobin), recorded allergies, weight and age of the patient, and cost of alternative treatments. Of course, for these decision support systems to achieve their greatest effects, clinicians need to interact with them by entering their orders themselves. This is more likely to occur in an academic health center, where house officers are expected to enter orders into the computer. These systems lead to more legible orders, fewer errors, and more thorough documentation of the reasons for orders, because clerks are not entering orders they must try to interpret from physicians' handwritten notes.

## Patient Education Systems

In the past five years, with the availability of inexpensive multimedia personal computers, many firms have created automated patient education systems. While patient education modules still appear on videotape and pamphlets more often than in digital form, patients prefer the interactive media of a personal computer. The computer can interact with and teach the patient according to instructions he or she has given it.

For instruction in dieting, management of hypertension and diabetes, reduction of stress, and management of AIDS, a system tailored to individual patients works best. Videotapes are viewed linearly, without variation or interaction. Computer programs can be much more engaging. Health risk assessments that patients complete on computers and that produce for each patient a specific set of instructions on how to change personal habits and reduce the likelihood of suffering specific chronic diseases are much more effective in changing patients' behavior than general purpose videos describing the consequences of bad habits for every man or woman.

Patients who complete structured educational sessions are better informed about their ailments, or their impending procedures; are more compliant with their treatments; are more likely to complete a course of therapy; require a shorter and less expensive postoperative recovery period; and use health care resources more prudently. One program, AskAdvice from First Data Corporation, produces instructional material about pharmaceuticals prescribed for patients. Patients appreciate the detailed documents, in layman's language, that the program provides.

## Physician Continuing Education Online

Computers can help physicians obtain continuing education in their offices and homes by using automated educational software and completing tests for CME credit online that may include management of simulated cases. The computer can test physicians' understanding of material it has just presented and accurately track the time a physician spends working on the system. Interactive continuing education via the Internet will become the next big opportunity for physicians to pursue their knowledge of new treatments and interpretations of patients' ailments. MedPartners has launched data-driven CME for its member physicians at www.medexcellence.com.

The Internet is a window on a much larger world, and the physician using it has access to millions of computers and users. Continuing education programs are available for credit without the physician's needing to install any software. Computers can store vast amounts of data, including images, on small optical CD-ROM disks and can access more data over the Internet, making continuing education more convenient and complete than that obtained from occasional sessions presented in the hospital and paid for by pharmaceutical firms.

The National Library of Medicine has funded the vast Visible Human project, of which the Visible Woman is more complete and more detailed than the Visible Man. For each project, a human cadaver has been serially sectioned in millimeter slices and imaged completely. All images are stored in digital format to allow three dimensional computer reconstruction of anatomic structures and organ systems. With these data, virtual reality training of physicians in anatomy will be much more thorough and accurate. The Visible Human is available on optical disks and via the Internet. There is now a magazine entitled the *Journal of Medicine and Virtual Reality*. It shows many ways in which virtual reality applications help clinicians learn how to perform surgery, understand anatomy, and visualize the distribution of metastatic malignancies.

## Telecommunication Technology

Telecommunication technology gives physicians access to computer-based medical records from a distance, any distance, and confidence that, when records are protected by encryption technology and passwords, people not intended to access them will be unable to do so. Communication with colleagues, health care facilities, pharmacies, utilization review firms, insurers, and public health services can be electronic, secure, and immediate. Many physicians already rely on electronic mail for their work. They communicate with colleagues on consultations and with facilities to schedule patients by e-mail.

Soon, e-mail will become multimedia, and physicians will send images, video, and sounds via e-mail for consultation requests to other physicians for second opinions. Teleradiology and telepathology already lend themselves to multimedia e-mail. Scheduling two physicians in a busy practice to participate in a simultaneous videoconference is difficult, but sending the same information by multimedia e-mail makes a lot of sense. It allows the sending physician to record a set of questions and store textual data and pertinent images about patients in question in a multimedia file, send it to a consultant, and wait for the consultant to check his or her electronic mail and download the file for interpretation.

As physicians obtain digital telephone service for electronic communication with ISDN and DSL, obtaining these large multimedia files will be much less time-consuming than it is now with modems operating at 57,600 bits per second. These faster digital telephone and cable connections are available in many urban areas now.

# Chapter 31
## Physician Executives Must Be Leaders in the Information Revolution

Why should physician executives care about medical informatics? Broadly defined, medical informatics is the study of the collection, storage, retrieval, and analysis of data and information in health care to support clinical and administrative decision making. Informatics is important because, in the past 10 years, powerful computer, software, and information technologies have been developed to enable health care organizations to automate some of the work of decision making for improved quality of care and cost control and for successful managed care contracting.

The technologies for collecting, storing, retrieving, and analyzing data (to produce information), information (to produce knowledge), and knowledge (to produce wisdom) are now almost entirely electronic and digital. Although informatics per se is a discipline independent of hardware and software and addresses the functional requirements for data in decision making, the technologies of digital information management still cost a lot of money, even though their performance-to-cost ratios continue to improve. These technologies are just beginning to affect directly the work of the most skilled knowledge workers in health care—physicians and nurses. They will become indispensable to them for decision support in the near future. The advent of practice guidelines will see to that.

Computer hardware and software have reached levels of performance that permit the creation of computer-based patient records. These devices can automate advice to clinicians about the care of individual patients and give clinicians the means of analyzing patterns of treatment for many patients, by many clinicians, in seconds. We have the means to replace paper records for health care services with electronic records and to bring the number-crunching power of computers to bear on the clinical data we place in electronic form. Even payers are demanding that providers produce more information about patients more quickly in electronic form. Regulators soon will expect that hospitals and health plans will have automated medical record systems in place before they grant them accreditation.

The technologies of computing and communication have already revolutionized the banking, financial services, travel, and airline industries. After the year 2000, they will revolutionize health care services as well and permit truly integrated health care systems to emerge. Computer-based patient records will move electronically over regional communication networks between locations of care and into physicians' homes and offices. Primary care services will be provided in patients' homes and consultative services in physicians' offices using telemedicine. Huge clinical databases will be available for quality improvement studies.

What is possible today—computer-based patient records, telemedicine, digital storage and electronic communication of x-rays, robotic fiberoptic surgery, voice recognition for dictation and order entry, radio-frequency local area networks and portable handheld computer terminals for nurses and physicians, and massive clinical databases and expert systems to survey them for opportunities for quality improvement—was not possible even a few years ago. And prices continue to plummet as the power of the technologies improves exponentially.

Until now, the principal assets of most health care organizations were the paper medical records of their patients. From now on, their principal assets will be computer-based patient records and the information and communication systems on which those records depend for their existence and transportation.

The investments necessary to stay apace of these technological developments are daunting, and the risks of selecting inadequate and incompatible information systems are great. Because technologies are changing so rapidly, the skills of most information systems staffs are not current. They tend to select information systems with older architectures (technologies) that they understand instead of newer systems with more modern architectures that may better meet the needs of their organizations, their affiliated clinicians, and patients in the future. Senior management teams must lead their organizations to select the best information and communication systems, working from a common knowledge base of current functional requirements for systems, of information technologies, and of technological trends.

Physician executives will lead their senior management teams to learn the state of the art in medical informatics and to share that common knowledge base. Physician executives will inherit the helm of integrated health care systems. They need to know how to invest wisely in these pervasive and transforming technologies. Informatics will be second only to clinical practice in importance as a discipline for a new generation of chief executives to comprehend when they take office, because successful information management will be the key to a competitive advantage for their organizations.

# Epilog

Soon patients, health plan members, and physicians will have inexpensive broadband communication networks entering their homes. Local telephone companies will offer DSL (digital subscriber line) service that uses a digital protocol to move bits over ordinary copper telephone wires at 1-5 megabits per second, depending on the protocol being used. Local cable television companies in many markets offer cable modems that give users access to up to 30 megabits per second per channel of bandwidth.

Soon, regulations implementing the Health Insurance Portability and Accountability Act of 1996 will be released by the National Committee of Vital and Health Statistics and adopted by the Department of Health and Human Services. The legislation calls for standardized electronic communication between providers and payers for claim submission, payment and remittance advice, enrollment and eligibility information, first report of injury, and referral certification and authorization. These steps will spare providers and payers some of the frustration and expense of communication for managed care that take place today by telephone, from clerk to clerk, or from clerk to clinician. Most significant will be the changes introduced by this sentence in the legislation: "The Secretary shall adopt standards providing for a standard unique health identifier for each individual, employer, health plan, and health care provider for use in the health care system."

With this sentence, Congress chose to assign every American a medical record number, instead of maintaining a system that expects a provider to assign a different number to each patient seen. The benefits of a single, unique medical record number for each American derive from our ability to integrate data from multiple locations of care to permit more reliable study of variation in health care services and outcomes over time. The cost to modify all health care transaction systems that assign numbers to patients, health plan members, and covered lives to accommodate these new personal identities will be substantial. Still, the potential benefits of learning from systematic clinical research activities outweigh the certain costs of modifying existing medical record numbering processes and the potential costs of breaches in patients' confidential information.

The HIPAA sets the stage for national electronic medical records, at last for simple administrative data from transactions of claims. The more difficult task of adopting a standardized nomenclature for clinical findings will evolve more slowly, abetted by the Unified Medical Language System (UMLS) project of the National Library of Medicine. Physicians and hospitals will build data warehouses to study their care retrospectively. The health evaluation sciences will flourish.

Health care informatics will attract clinicians inclined to electronics and computing to lead the digitization of medical records and implementation of digital informatics management systems. Managed care will evolve to managing care, and clinicians well-informed in health care informatics will lead.

## Conclusion

Digital electronic systems are here to stay. Technologies for digital capture and storage of information will continue to improve over the next several decades. We will learn to standardize the information we use to describe our patients, and all of us, patients and providers of care, will benefit from the analysis of digital information about our patients.

# Glossary

## A

**Active Storage:** Auxiliary memory dedicated to data that have long-term value and must be accessed easily and quickly. Commonly found on floppy or hard disks.

**Address:** The computer designation for a particular cell of memory and its contents.

**ADP:** Automatic data processing.

**AHDMS:** Automated hospital data management system.

**AHIS:** Automated hospital information system.

**AI:** Artificial intelligence.

**AIDSLINE:** On-line MEDLARS database on AIDS.

**AIDSTRIALS:** On-line MEDLARS database on AIDS drugs.

**American Standard Code Information Exchange (ASCII):** A seven-bit code for the exchange of alphanumeric data among data processing and data communication equipment. May be referred to as "unformatted." (See EBCDIC.)

**AMIA:** American Medical Informatics Association.

**AMRS:** Automated medical record system.

**Analog Data:** Presentation of information exactly as it originally occurs or is measured. For instance, a telephone transmission is an analog presentation of the original voice data. (See digital data.)

**Analog-to-Digital Conversion:** A process or device by which analog data are translated into digital form.

**Application Program:** Instructions to the computer for handling specific user projects or applications, such as accounting, word processing, inventory control, medical records, and the like.

**Architecture:** The design of a computer's internal operations—directories, memory, programs, input/output structure, etc. Also, the design of the computer with regard to all peripheral devices—printers, modems, etc.

**Archival Storage:** Use of hard disk and magnetic tape for the retention of information for long-term use. Commonly used for back-up, documentary, and legal data.

**Artificial Intelligence (AI):** Simulation by computers of human reasoning and learning functions.

**ASCII:** American Standard Code for Information Exchange.

**Assembler:** A program that translates assembly-language programs into machine-language programs.

**Assembly Language:** Low-level mnemonic instructions for communication with computers.

**Attribute Data:** Classification or accounting of events, items, or units on the basis of their quality characteristics. Data are usually expressed as whole numbers on a discrete scale of measurement.

**Automated Patient Record:** Immediate placement of medical record information into computer form. In purest form, eliminates need for paper record altogether. Provides for retrieval of data from multiple locations and ability to extract data for quality indicators.

**Auxiliary Memory:** Hard disks, floppy disks, and magnetic tape storage of information or programs not needed in main memory.

# B

**Bandwidth:** In the transmission of information, the amount of data in bits that can be transmitted per unit of time.

**Baseband:** Transmission of information in which a single, unmodulated stream of data is involved.

**Batch Mode:** Control of computer usage by a central staff, to which users send projects and then wait for results. The process may involve remote transmission, whereby projects are transmitted by modem to the central point.

**Batch Program:** Method of processing of groups of data that have been collected over time or that must be accounted for periodically.

**Baud Rate:** The speed at which data are transmitted, expressed in bits per second.

*Glossary*

**BCD:** Binary-coded decimal.

**Biotechnology:** An applied biological science, such as bioengineering, or its products, such as recombinant DNA technology.

**Bit Map:** The digital representation of an image or a graphic in memory. The memory bits have a one-on-one correspondence with the image or graphic pixels on the monitor screen.

**Bit:** An electronic switch in computer memory that assumes a value of 0 or 1 (off or on). All alphanumeric data in computer memory are constructed from bits and bytes.

**Boot:** To start a computer so that its operational programs are loaded and available for use.

**Booting:** See bootstrap.

**Bootstrap:** A set of instructions that is permanently installed in the computer's read only memory and that is used each time the computer is turned on. Execution of the bootstrap is called booting the computer.

**BPS:** Bits per second.

**Broadband:** Transmission of information in which data signals are modulated within a frequency range and several signals can be accommodated in the same transmission.

**Browse:** Feature of many database application programs by which files may be scanned for information of interest.

**Buffer:** An area of memory used to temporarily store data being transferred from one computer hardware device to another, such as data awaiting processing by a printer. Buffers are used to compensate for variations in the rates at which devices process data.

**Bus Network:** A system by which linked computer workstations communicate through a common information distribution channel.

**Byte:** A grouping of eight bits processed by the computer as a unit. Bytes are the building blocks for characters in computer language.

# C

**CAD:** Computer-assisted diagnosis, computer-assisted design.

**CAI:** Computer-assisted instruction.

**CD-ROM:** Off-line method of storing computer based information and files. The Compact Disc-Read Only Memory is capable of storing very large amounts of information, including complex graphical presentations.

**Cell:** The storage dimension for a single unit of information, such as a bit, a byte, or a word. Also the location of a single entry of data in a computer spreadsheet.

**Central Processing Unit:** Hardware and associated resident program instructions that control interpretation and execution of all other instructions to the computer. Sometimes called the "brain" of the computer.

**Central System:** A single computer system that satisfies all of an organization's computing needs through use of common databases and interfaces.

**Checksheet:** A data recording form that indicates how many times things have happened.

**CHIN:** Community health information network.

**Chip:** An electronic device that contains the circuitry and components that perform the computer's functions and serve as its memory.

**Clinical Decision Making:** The process by which the clinician gathers data on a patient and his or her condition and arrives at a diagnosis, treatment program, and prognosis.

**Clustering Techniques:** A variety of approaches used to find patterns within sets of data.

**COBOL:** Common Business-Oriented Language for computers.

**Combobox:** A format commonly used in database data entry forms that constrains the user to a specific set of choices.

**Command:** A user-generated computer instruction.

**Compact Disc-Read Only Memory (CD-ROM):** Laser-based technology that permits the recording of large amounts of data on a single disk for later multiple readings by computer.

**Compiler:** A program that translates high-level programming language (human language and symbols) into machine language.

**Computer-Aided Instruction (CAI):** The application of computers to educational programming.

**Computer-Assisted Design (CAD):** Use of computers and computer programs for image-driven, graphical fine-tuning of physical designs through a real-time trial-and-error process.

**Computerized Medical Record:** See automated medical record.

*Glossary*

**Contrast Resolution:** The number of bits per pixel in a graphic computer display. Used to measure the ability to distinguish screen or print-out intensity levels.

**Control Chart:** A graphic representation of a process over time that consists of a map of collected data on the process and the establishment of upper and lower control limits on the process. When the data collected on the process fall outside the control limits, the process is said to be out of control.

**Core Memory:** Random-access portion of main memory that can be accessed directly by the central processing unit.

**Crash:** Accidental or catastrophic shutdown of a computer due to hardware or user error.

**Cursor:** A blinking or otherwise highlighted indicator on the monitor screen of where the next character is to appear, where a correction is to be placed, or where the next piece of information is to be placed.

**Custom-Designed:** A computer system whose hardware and software are specific to the organization in which they are used.

**Cut and Paste:** A technique in many word processing and graphic application programs by which groups of words or images can be moved intact to a new location.

# D

**Database:** A collection of stored data and the organizational logic of their storage pattern.

**Database Management System (DBMS):** The set of programs that provides access to and allows manipulation of databases.

**Data Bus:** A system that connects the central processing unit, data storage elements, and all peripheral devices for the exchange of data within a computer system.

**Data Management:** All of the functions necessary for the computerized organizing, cataloging, locating, retrieving, storing, and maintaining of data.

**dBase:** A popular commercial database management software package that allows access to multiple files in the database simultaneously and design of screen fields that are user-specific.

**Debugger:** A system program that allows programmers to locate and correct errors in programming.

**Decision Support System:** Generally used to describe computer-based data acquisition and analysis systems used to make clinical decisions about patients' conditions.

**Decision Tree:** In clinical decision making, the process of moving from a general diagnosis to more and more specific evaluation of the patient's injury or condition. A graphic presentation of an algorithm.

**Desktop Computer:** A complete computer system, including all peripheral units, that fits on a desktop. Commonly used to describe computerized production of printed and published materials.

**Digital Data:** Information expressed in the form of numerical digits.

**Directory:** In a computer, the partition of operating system and data files into distinct collections. Also used to describe the index of these files. Directories may be further divided into a hierarchy of subdirectories for both volume and logic reasons. Directories and subdirectories of computer files are equivalent to physical filing cabinets or cabinet drawers.

**Disk.** A magnetic device for storage of information and programs for computers.

**Distributed System:** A collection of independent computers that share data, programs, and other resources, such as printers, scanners, modems, and other peripheral components.

**Document:** See file.

**DOS (Disk Operating System).** A specialized program, installed in main memory during booting, that provides a link between the user and the computer's disk drives, both floppy and hard.

**Dot Matrix Printer:** A printer that creates characters and graphics by imposition of dot patterns. The quality of printing is determined by the number of dots used in each print field. This technology has largely given way to laser and other more advanced printing technqiues.

**Download:** Process of transferring data or programs from a computer to another computer, to a storage medium, to a printer, or to any other device.

**Drive:** Hardware components necessary for transferring data to and from a floppy disk.

**Driver:** Software instructions that the computer follows to format data for transfer to printers and other peripheral devices.

**Digital Subscriber Line (DSL):** A digital protocol from the telephone company for moving digital data over copper telephone wire at 1-5 million bits per second.

**Dumb Terminal:** A visual display terminal and keyboard with minimal input/output capability and no processing capability.

**Dynamic Data Exchange (DDE):** An established protocol for exchanging data through active links between applications that run under Microsoft Windows®.

# E

**EGA (Enhanced Graphics Adapter):** A display technology for the PC; it has now been replaced by VGA.

**Electronic Data Interchange (EDI):** A protocol for creating common data definitions for the purpose of exchanging business-related data elements.

**Electronic Patient Record:** See automated patient record.

**Electronic Mail:** The process of sending, receiving, storing, and forwarding messages between users on a telecommunications or local area network.

**Electronic Spreadsheet:** A program typically operated on a personal computer that is used to facilitate budgeting or financial planning.

**Epidemiological Analysis:** Use of traditional epidemiological techniques to measure outcomes in given populations and thus determine the effectiveness of care (i.e., observational studies such as cohort studies or case-control studies).

**Erase:** The removal of data or commands from a computer record.

**External Coded Decimal Interchange Code (EBCDIC):** An 8-bit computer code used to represent data. It is the principal code now used in computers and can represent up to 256 distinct characters.

# F

**Field:** A single piece of information, the smallest unit manipulated by a database management system. Also, the series of positions on the computer monitor occupied by the information—for instance, an address.

**File:** A repository of computer data (e.g., a word processing document) or of program instruction (e.g., winword.exe).

**Floppy Disk:** A flexible disk of oxide-coated mylar used for the storage of data. Most common sizes are 5¼" and 3½". The disk is inserted in the computer drive for data manipulation and processing.

**Flow Chart:** A diagram of a process, showing each step of the process and how it relates to other steps.

**Flowsheet:** Tabular presentation of information in a format that permits display of variables that change with time. Also, the software that permits manipulation of the information.

**Font:** A complete set of characters in a particular typeface style and size.

# G

**Graphic User Interface (GUI):** Computer control system that allows the user to command the computer by "pointing and clicking," using a mouse, at icons or pictures representing applications or files in computer memory.

**Graphic:** A picture or illustration generated by a computer and displayed on screen, paper, or film. Requires special computers and computer hardware.

**Gray Scale:** A computer scheme for representing intensity within a black-and-white image. Involves use of varying bits per graphics pixel.

# H

**Hard Disk:** Hardware for auxiliary storage of large amounts of data. May be a separate device or be located within the computer.

**Hardware:** The physical components of a computer, such as central processing unit, keyboard, monitor, printer, modem, and data storage devices.

**HIS:** Hospital information system, health information system.

**HISSG:** Hospital information system sharing group.

**Histogram:** A pictorial or graphic summary of a set of data to highlight patterns.

**HMSS:** Hospital Management Systems Society.

# I

**Icon:** An on-screen graphic that may be used to access programs, data files, commands, or other stored or computer-embedded information.

# Glossary

**Impact Printer:** A data output device that imprints through contact of raised type against paper, using ink or ribbon as the transfer medium.

**Informatics:** The whole of information technology and its applications.

**Information Science:** The study of creation, use, and communication of information.

**Information Sharing:** Comparison of physician practice patterns and/or performance and cost information provided by HMOs and hospitals for sharing with consumers.

**Information System:** Equipment and procedures used for the collection, recording, processing, storage, retrieval, and display of information.

**Information Theory:** The mathematical formulations that explain the communication of information.

**Input Device:** Hardware, such as a keyboard, a mouse, or a light pen, used to enter data into a computer.

**Installation:** The process by which software programs are stored on a computer.

**Instruction:** Coding that defines an operation that is requested of a computer.

**Intelligent Terminal:** An input/output device in which computer processing components are built into the terminal.

**Interface:** The physical (connector or keyboard) or logical (software) link between the computer and a user or peripheral device (printer, modem, etc.).

**Internet:** International computer communications system and protocols that links computers and computer networks.

**Interpreter:** An internal computer translator that converts source language into machine language.

**Intranet:** A computer-based information sharing system within a single organization.

# J

**Joystick:** Electromechanical device that is used to move the computer cursor. Usually used with video games.

## K

**Keyboard:** Electromechanical alphanumeric device for typing program commands and data for a computer.

**Key Field:** Coding within a record that uniquely identifies a record within a file.

**Knowledge Base:** The database of facts, inferences, and procedures needed for problem solving on a particular subject.

## L

**LAN:** Local area network.

**Laser:** Light amplification by stimulated emission of radiation.

**Laser Printer:** A nonimpact output device that uses laser technology for transfer of data images to paper.

**Light Pen:** Photosensitive device used in conjunction with the monitor and software to provide data and program commands.

**Literature Search:** Use of software program that permits key word scanning of literature databases for articles and books on selected topics.

**Local Area Network (LAN):** Linked computers and software programs that permit sharing of data and peripheral devices by multiple users in a single site.

## M

**Machine Language:** The basic language of a computer requiring no further translation.

**Macro:** A single source language statement that, when translated, results in a series of machine-language statements.

**Magnetic Tape:** A data storage device, usually in a cassette.

**Mainframe:** Large computers with large amounts of storage capacity and the ability to process large amounts of data very quickly.

# Glossary 213

**Management Information Systems:** Equipment and procedures used for the collection, recording, processing, storage, retrieval, and display of information relevant to an organization.

**Maser:** Microwave amplification by stimulated emission of radiation.

**Medical Computer Science:** The branch of computer science that deals with medical applications.

**Medical Informatics:** Study of the management and use of biomedical information.

**Medical Information Science:** See medical informatics.

**Medical Information Systems:** Any equipment or procedures used for the collection, recording, processing, storage, retrieval, and display of clinical information.
**Medical Record:** The format, sometimes electronic, in which all information on a patient and his or her encounters with a health care organization are recorded. Refers to the individual encounter and to the sum of an individual's encounters with the organization.

**Medical Records Review:** See medical audit.

**Medlars:** Medical Literature Analysis and Retrieval System.

**Medline:** A literature database on medical sciences and health care management topics maintained by the National Library of Medicine. Medlars on line.

**Memory:** Areas of the computer that are used for storage of data and software program.

**Menu:** A list of options from which the user may select programs or program elements.

**Menu-Driven:** A software program that is operated through selection from a series of menu options.

**MeSH:** Medical subject headings.

**Microcomputer:** The smallest and least expensive computers, these devices use microprocessors as their central processing units.

**Microprocessor:** The basic control devices for microcomputers and other small computer devices, these integrated circuit chips contain the arithmetic, logic, and control elements required for data processing.

**Minicomputer:** The midrange of computers, fitting in size, cost, and complexity between microcomputers and mainframes.

**MIS:** Management information system.

**Modem (Modulator-Demodulator):** A peripheral device that translates computer digital data into analog signals for telephone transmission to external computers and computer-driven devices.

**Modular System:** A computer system composed of separate units, each of which performs a specific set of functions.

**Monitor:** The video display unit of a computer workstation.

**Mouse:** A device that works with software programs to move data or other objects on the monitor screen, to select from menu options, and generally to operate the cursor.

**Multiprocessing:** The simultaneous processing of two or more sets of instructions by multiple central processing units under common control.

**Multiprogramming:** Shared and simultaneous operation of two or more programs by a single computer.

# N

**Network Topology:** The configuration of the physical connections in a computer communication network.

**Node:** A terminal, station, communication computer, or other device in a network.

**Noise:** Any unwanted, spurious, or otherwise unintended signal in a device or system.

# O

**Object-Oriented Program:** A programming technique that uses computer code to produce reusable objects that act in a definable way rather than the traditional method of computer code that defines instructions for acting upon a data element.

**OLE (Object Linking and Embedding):** The process by which an object from one computer application may be shared with another, eliminating the need to recreate the object. This technology allows changing of the new object to update the old.

**On-line:** Connected to and communicating directly with the computer's central processing unit.

**Operating System:** Software that controls the execution of computer programs and provides numerous housekeeping, accounting, and data management services.

# Glossary

**Optical Character Reader:** An input device that reads characters on printed documents by their shapes, translating them into machine language for further manipulation.

**Optical Disk.** A high-density storage device that uses laser technology.

**Output Device:** Printers, plotters, and other units for display of computer data.

# P

**Parallel Processing:** Simultaneous execution of two or more processes in multiple devices.

**Patient Profile:** Computer-based summary of key medical and demographic information on a given patient.

**PERT:** Program evaluation and review technique.

**Peripheral Device:** Printers, modems, FAX equipment, plotters, hard drives, and other devices connected to the central processing unit for the translation and/or transmission of data into more usable form.

**Personal Computer:** A moderately priced microcomputer intended for personal rather than business use. (See microcomputer.)

**Pixel:** The smallest unit on the monitor screen that can be stored, displayed, or addressed. The building block for computer graphics.

**Point-of-Care System:** A hospital information system that includes bedside terminals for the acquisition and storage of patient data.

**POMR:** Problem-oriented medical record.

**Primary Data:** Information specifically collected to solve a current problem. Raw or original data collected during the delivery of care.

**Printer:** An output device that produces hard copies of computer data.

**Private Branch Exchange (PBX):** A telephone switching center.

**Program Language:** A formal language by which computer programs are specified for the computer hardware.

**Program:** A series of instructions that cause the computer to process data in a prescribed manner.

**Prompt:** A message from the computer that it is ready to accept the prescribed data or command.

# Q

**QBE (Query by Example):** A method of selecting various elements from a database, defining limits for these elements, and using them to sort through the database to create a report.

**Query:** A request for specific information from the computer.

**Queue:** An ordered list of jobs waiting for computer or peripheral unit execution.

# R

**Random-Access Memory (RAM):** The working memory of the computer, into which programs are loaded and then executed.

**Raster Scan:** A pattern of rows of dots on a monitor that form an image.

**Read Only Memory (ROM):** The portion of the computer's memory that can be read but that cannot be written into. This is the permanent portion of the computer memory.

**Real Time:** Data management and manipulation at the same time that it is entered into the computer.

**Record:** A grouping of data fields in a file that refers to information about a single entity.

**Register:** A group of electronic switches in a computer that are used to store and manipulate data.

**Resolution:** The amount of information that a video display can reproduce, expressed by the number of pixels in the display. High-resolution displays are smooth and realistic; low-resolution displays are jagged and blocky.

# S

**Sampling Rate:** The rate at which the value of an analog signal is measured and recorded.

# Glossary

**Scan:** The process by which a picture, illustration, or document is examined to produce an image on a monitor screen or an image file in a computer.

**Scanner:** An optical device that recognizes a specified set of visual symbols.

**Schema:** The overall organization of a database.

**Screen:** The visual display portion of a computer monitor.

**Scroll Bar:** An element of a graphic user interface screen that allows the user to "scroll" down through a list of elements or down a page of data.

**Server:** A central device in a computer network that connects individual devices and users to the central processing unit for the network.

**Situational Analysis:** An informal study of information already available in the problem area.

**Software.** The programs or instructions that instruct a computer. Software may be built into the computer's ROM or loaded as needed from disk or tape.

**Soundex:** A search mechanism that permits looking up a "text" name by selecting the first few consonants of text to find potential homonyms and misspellings.

**Spatial Resolution:** A measure of the ability to distinguish on a monitor screen between proximate points.

**Spreadsheet:** A software program that organizes data and formulas into a matrix of cells.

**Star Network:** A computer network configuration in which individual workstations are arranged in parallel.

**Storage:** A device or medium that can accept, hold, and deliver data on demand.

**Structured Query Language (SQL):** A standardized language used for querying, updating, and managing relational databases.

**Subdirectory:** A collection of files packaged in a directory that is contained within a larger directory of files and other subdirectories.

**Syntax:** The rules that govern the structure of a computer language and its expressions. The computer issues an error message when language syntax is violated.

**System:** Any group of related processes intended to achieve a specific outcome.

**System Program:** Software program that governs the internal operations of the computer. See application program.

**Systems Theory:** Principles, models, and laws that apply to complex interrelationships and interdependencies of sets of linked components that form a functioning whole and that themselves may be systems.

# T

**Tab:** A carriage control that specifies output columns.

**TAG:** Technical advisory group.

**Technological Imperative:** An obligation to apply technology to the body of scientific knowledge wherever possible.

**Technology Assessment:** The systematic and scientific evaluation of the cost- and risk-effectiveness of both existing and new forms of technology.

**Telemedicine:** The provision of medical diagnosis and consulting services by long-distance electronic means.

**Temporal Resolution:** The amount of time between acquisition by the computer of each of a series of images.

**Terminal:** The collection of devices used to input data and programs to the computer and to receive output from the computer.

**Text Editor:** A software program for the preparation and manipulation of written material.

**Text Scanner:** A device for the translation of printed documents into computer language.

**Time-Share Mode:** Simultaneous operation of a computer by several users. Because of the speed of computers, what is actually sequential access appears to be simultaneous.

**Touch Screen:** A monitor screen on which commands can be entered by pressing designated areas with a finger or other object.

**Turnkey:** A prepackaged computer system containing all the hardware, software, training, and maintenance needed for a given application.

# U

**Universal Product Code (UPC):** Special identifying marks (bar code) for each product readable by electronic scanners.

*Glossary*

**UNIX:** A powerful computer operating system with many high-level utility programs that is capable of running a number of jobs simultaneously.

**Upload:** To transfer user data to a remote computer system. To transfer data from a disk or other storage device to a computer.

**Utilization Data:** Information collected on physician practice patterns.

# V

**Validity:** The extent to which data measure what they are intended to measure.

**VGA (Video Graphics Array):** Standard PC display standard that provides medium resolution for text and graphics.

**Video Display Terminal:** A monitor and keyboard for computer input and output.

**Virtual Memory:** The use of auxiliary data storage units as if they were computer memory.

**Voice Recognition:** Direct conversion of spoken data into computer language.

**Voxel:** The smallest unit of a three-dimensional computer image. (See pixel.)

# W

**Wide-Area Network:** A network that connects computers dispersed over a large geographic area.

**Wild Card:** A computer technique that allows performance of utility functions on multiple files with similar names. Commonly involves the use of an asterisk or some other code as the wild card designation.

**Windows®:** A powerful operating system that allows monitor display of two or more programs simultaneously.

**Word Processing:** Any of several software programs for writing, revising, manipulating, formatting, and printing text for letters, reports, manuscripts, and other printed matter.

**Word Wrapping:** A word processing technique that automatically moves a word to the next line if it doesn't fit at the end of the original line.

**Word:** A sequence of bits that are accessed in memory as a unit.

**Workstation:** A configuration of computer equipment and peripheral devices that are intended for use by a single person.

**WORM (Write Once Read Many):** A technology for recording data on optical media in such a way that they cannot be edited or overwritten but can be read multiple times.

**WYSIWYG (What You See Is What You Get):** In word processing programs, screen images—typefaces, format, etc.—that appear exactly as they will in the printed document.